Pocket Picture Guides
to Clinical Medicine

Sexually Transmitted Diseases

Pocket Picture Guides
to Clinical Medicine

Sexually Transmitted Diseases

James S. Bingham TD, MB, BCh, BAO, MRCOG

Consultant in Genito-Urinary Medicine,
The Middlesex Hospital, London, UK .

Williams & Wilkins Baltimore London

Western Hemisphere distribution rights held by
Williams and Wilkins
428 East Preston Street
Baltimore, MD 21202, USA

ISBN 0-906923-16-6 (Gower)
       0-683-00915-X (Williams and Wilkins)

Library of Congress Cataloging in Publication Data
Bingham, J.
            Sexually transmitted diseases.
            (Pocket picture guides to clinical medicine)
            1. Venereal diseases-Diagnosis-Atlases. I. Title
II. Series. [DNLM: 1. Venereal diseases-Diagnosis-Atlases.
WC 17 B613s]
RC200.5.B56 1984b   616.95′1075   83-5765

Project Editor: Fiona Carr
    Designer: Teresa Foster

Originated in Hong Kong by Imago Publishing Ltd.
Printed in Great Britain by W. S. Cowell Ltd.

Pocket Picture Guides
to Clinical Medicine

The purpose of this series is to provide essential visual information about commonly encountered diseases in a convenient practical and economic format. Each Pocket Picture Guide covers an important area of day-to-day clinical medicine. The main feature of these books is the superbly photographed colour reproductions of typical clinical appearances. Other visual diagnostic information, such as X-rays, is included where appropriate. Each illustration is fully explained by a clearly written descriptive caption highlighting important diagnostic features. Tables presenting other diagnostic and differential diagnostic information are included where appropriate. A comprehensive and carefully compiled index makes each Pocket Picture Guide an easy to use source of visual reference.

An extensive series is planned and other titles in the initial group of Pocket Picture Guides are:

Infectious Diseases
Rheumatic Diseases
Skin Diseases
Pediatrics

Acknowledgements
Most of the pictures in this book are taken from the
departmental collection at James Pringle House, The
Middlesex Hospital, built up over the years by the
medical staff of the department but mainly by Dr. R. D.
Catterall. I am indebted to him for permitting
reproduction of the pictures. The following have also
kindly given permission for their photographs to be
reproduced (and I apologise for any omissions): Professor
M. W. Adler, Dr. Anona Blackwell, Professor I. McL.
Brown, Dr. E. M. C. Dunlop, Dr. H. L. Gardner, Dr. A.
Latif, Dr. A. G. Lawrence, Dr. G. M. Levene, Dr. J. A.
McCutchan, Dr. A. Mindel, Mr. M. Newman, Dr. C. S.
Nicol, Dr. Elisabeth Rees, Dr. Sheena Sutherland and
Dr. R. R. Willcox. Dr. C. S. Nicol's slides are reproduced
by permission of Baillière Tindall.

Some of the conditions depicted are seen only rarely in
the UK today, and so it has not always been possible to
provide high quality pictures in every case (for example
Figs. 95 and 96).

Contents

Introduction   1

Urethral discharge   3
    Non-specific urethritis (NSU)   5
    Reiter's disease   7
    Gonorrhoea   12

Vaginal discharge   19
    Candidosis   21
    Trichomoniasis   24
    Gardnerella-associated discharge   26
    Non-specific cervicitis   27
    Gonococcal cervicitis   30

Genital ulceration   33
    Herpes   35
    Primary syphilis   40
    Secondary syphilis   49
    Late forms of syphilis   64
    Congenital syphilis   72
    Chancroid   76
    Lymphogranuloma venereum   80
    Granuloma inguinale   84

Genital warts, molluscum contagiosum, infestations and Kaposi's sarcoma   87
    Warts   88
    Infestations   95
    Molluscum contagiosum   98
    Kaposi's sarcoma   99

Index

Introduction

The sexually transmitted diseases (STDs) have increased
dramatically in incidence over the last 25 years, all over the
world. Between 1960 and 1980 the number of new cases
attending STD clinics increased by a factor of four in
England and Wales. Whereas 50 years ago syphilis,
gonorrhoea and chancroid were the main STDs recognised,
since the Second World War it has been realised that many
other diseases are sexually transmissible. In the last 10 years
the spectrum of disease transmissible by sexual contact has
further widened with the recognition of infections
transmitted predominantly between homosexual men,
namely hepatitis B and enteric infections spread as a result
of oro-anal contact, hepatitis A, amoebiasis and giardiasis.
Recently the acquired immune deficiency syndrome (AIDS),
mostly seen in homosexual men and frequently resulting in
death, has been the cause of increasing concern particularly
as the aetiology and means of transmission is as yet
unknown.

   This book does not pretend to give a comprehensive
coverage of all the STDs, firstly because it is small and
secondly because not all the conditions lend themselves to
photographic representation. Illustrations of the non-
sexually transmitted diseases mentioned are not included.
No attempt has been made to include details of treatment of
the conditions, as this changes from time to time and will
vary from place to place. It must necessarily be read,
therefore, in conjunction with a standard textbook on the
subject.

   In the interests of simplicity the book has been divided
into sections, each representing the complaints that might
bring patients along to seek advice. This means that syphilis,
for instance, will appear under genital ulceration, although
many of the photographs of the different stages of the disease
will not represent ulceration. Gonorrhoea in the male will
appear under urethral discharge but, in the female, it will be
included in the section on vaginal discharge. It is hoped that
this problem-orientated approach will prove helpful.

1

Conditions which are sexually transmitted or which may be transmissible as a result of sexual activity

Non-specific genital infection
Gonorrhoea
Genital warts
Genital candidosis
Trichomoniasis
Genital herpes
Syphilis
Tropical STDs:
       Chancroid
       Lymphogranuloma venereum
       Granuloma inguinale

Skin infestations:
       Scabies
       Pediculosis pubis

Molluscum contagiosum

Diseases predominantly spread between homosexual men:
       Hepatitis B
       Enteric infection: Hepatitis A
                       Amoebiasis
                       Giardiasis
                       ? AIDS
Cytomegalovirus infection

Urethral discharge

Discharge from the urethra is the commonest presenting symptom in men seen at STD departments. Pathological discharge must be distinguished from discharge of physiological origins such as crystalluria (a chalky discharge at the end of micturition), prostatorrhoea (discharge during defaecation), and secretion due to sexual arousal.

It is important to differentiate between subpreputial discharge, such as physiologically produced smegma and balanoposthitis due for instance to candidal infection, and actual urethral discharge.

Profuse, purulent discharge is likely to be due to gonorrhoea and less profuse mucoid, white discharge is more likely to be due to non-specific urethritis. However, it is not possible to determine the aetiology of urethral discharge by inspection alone. As a first step a Gram-stained smear of the urethral discharge should be made. Where urethritis exists polymorphonuclear leucocytes will be seen. If these contain Gram-negative intracellular diplococci a presumptive diagnosis of gonorrhoea can be made which can later be confirmed by culture. Where no evidence of gonorrhoea is found the patient has non-gonococcal urethritis. A small number of these cases can be due to trichomonal infection, a few to candidal and herpetic infections (although there is usually other visible evidence of these conditions on the glans penis) and, occasionally, a chemical urethritis can be produced by instillation of strong solutions into the urethra. Intrameatal and intraurethral lesions such as warts and urethral stricture may sometimes be associated with a discharge. Other bacteria such as *Escherichia coli*, *Klebsiella* and *Proteus* can rarely produce urethritis in diabetic, immunocompromised or debilitated patients but, if none of these causes is readily identifiable, the patient is assumed to have non-specific urethritis (NSU).

Aetiology of urethral discharge

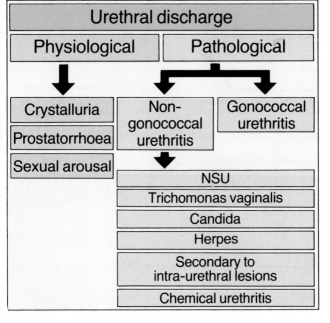

NSU is the commonest cause of urethral discharge in the Western World. Its aetiology is not fully known, but about half of the cases are believed to be due to *Chlamydia trachomatis*. Its incubation period is usually between 6 and 14 days and may be as long as 6 weeks. The incubation period in gonorrhoea is much shorter, generally between 2 and 6 days. Since the advent of the antibiotic era, in developed countries where patients usually seek treatment early, complications of both these conditions are rare.

Non-specific urethritis (NSU)

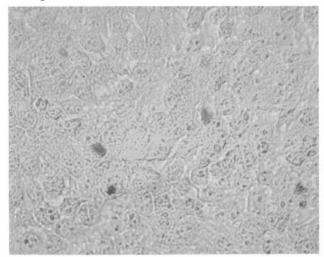

Fig. 1 *Chlamydia trachomatis* of the subtypes D-K may be found in about 50% of cases of non-specific genital infection. A bacterium and obligate intracellular parasite, it cannot be grown on ordinary culture media, and requires to be grown on tissue culture. Here, chlamydial inclusions on tissue culture are seen stained with iodine.

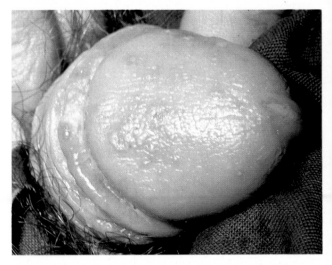

Fig. 2 Urethral 'discharge' in NSU may range from meatal moistness to a purulent discharge. Most cases, however, have a translucent white discharge. In this case, there is meatitis and also pouting of the meatus. Note too the balanoposthitis.

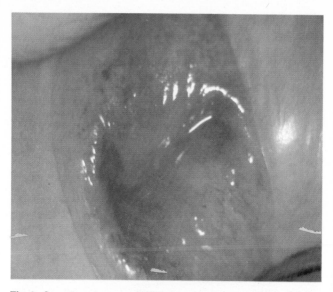

Fig. 3 Sometimes in cases of NSU, there may be only minimal urethral discharge, but considerable meatitis may co-exist; in this case it is associated with chlamydial infection.

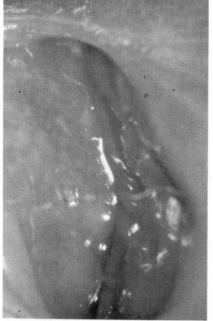

Fig. 4 In long-standing cases of urethritis due to *Chlamydia trachomatis,* follicles may occasionally be visible at the urethral meatus.

Reiter's disease

Reiter's disease may occur following a dysenteric illness and in association with non-gonococcal urethritis in less than 1% of cases.

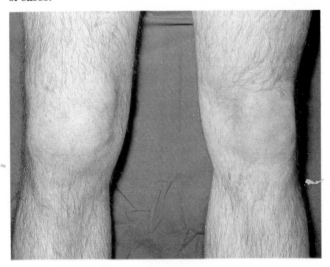

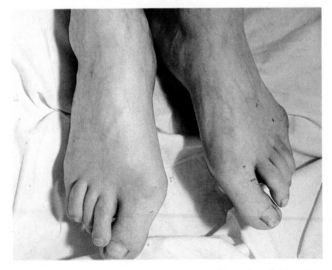

Fig. 5 The majority of cases present with arthritis (and tendinitis and fasciitis) and this is usually the dominant clinical feature. It may be associated with constitutional upset. There is often a predilection for the knee, ankle, foot and sacroiliac joints. In these pictures the right knee and right first metatarsophalangeal joints are affected.

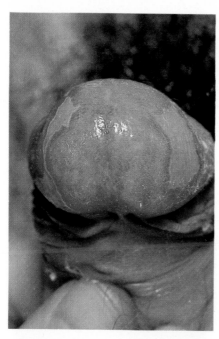

Fig. 6 Circinate balanitis occurs in 20% of cases of Reiter's disease, particularly in the uncircumcised. Small erosions may become confluent and develop a raised circinate margin.

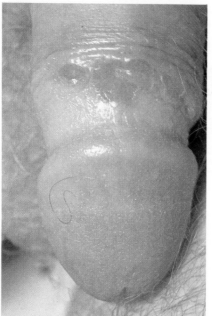

Fig. 7 The undersurface of the retracted prepuce may also become eroded and this can extend to the glans. As the condition settles down, so too does the erosion, and topical steroid therapy is generally not helpful.

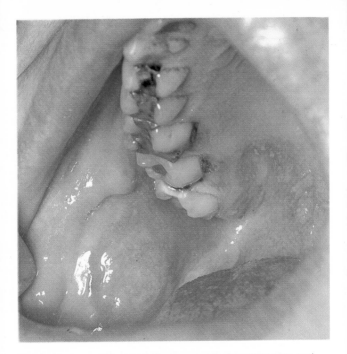

Fig. 8 Mucous erosions may also occur on the buccal mucosa, and occasionally on the tongue in Reiter's disease. The lesions are not generally painful and resolve spontaneously as the activity of the condition subsides.

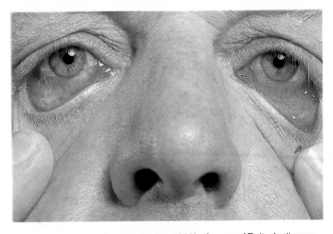

Fig. 9 The eyes are involved in about 30% of cases of Reiter's disease. Conjunctivitis is the commonest problem. One or both eyes may be affected and it is usually most marked at the lateral angles.

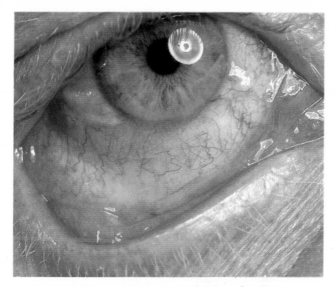

Fig. 10 Considerable conjunctival oedema may occur. When the disease flares up, so too does the conjunctivitis and it settles as the attack subsides. Severe cases may be helped by steroid drops.

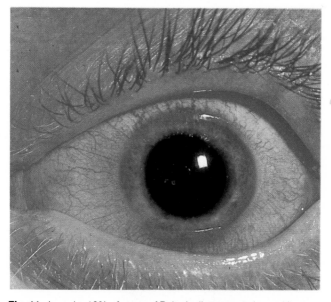

Fig. 11 In under 10% of cases of Reiter's disease anterior uveitis may occur. This is a serious complication and requires expert ophthalmological management. Relapses are common.

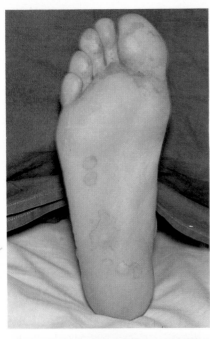

Fig. 12 In about 15% of cases, erythematous macules may appear on the soles of the feet, developing into pustules and later becoming hyperkeratotic. This is known as keratoderma blennorrhagica. It may occasionally be found elsewhere on the skin, particularly on the legs and scalp.

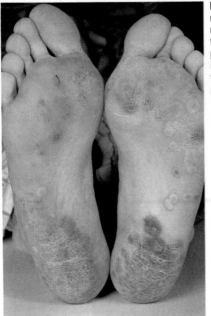

Fig. 13 The lesions may increase in number and coalesce to form thick crusted plaques. The condition is histologically similar to certain types of pustular psoriasis.

11

Gonorrhoea

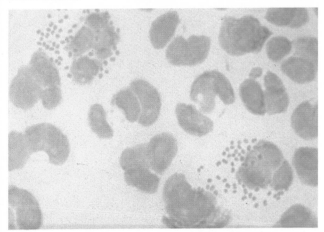

Fig. 14 The causative organism is *Neisseria gonorrhoeae*. A smear made from the urethral discharge should be Gram stained. Pus cells will be seen and, if gonorrhoea is the cause of the discharge, intracellular Gram-negative diplococci will be visible. In female patients detection on a smear is not as easy and the diagnosis is often only made by culturing the organism.

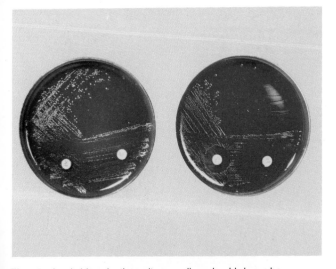

Fig. 15 A suitable selective culture medium should always be inoculated in order to confirm the diagnosis. Fluorescein staining methods and sugar fermentation tests are then used to identify the gonococcus. Ideally, antibiotic sensitivity tests should be carried out on all strains, and here penicillin discs are employed.

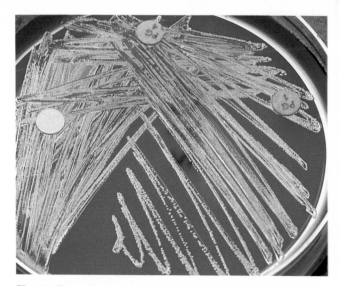

Fig. 16 The penicillinase-producing gonococcus was first identified in 1976. It is now particularly prevalent in South East Asia and in West Africa, but is generally increasing in incidence throughout the world. Here, such a strain is seen to be unaffected by penicillin discs.

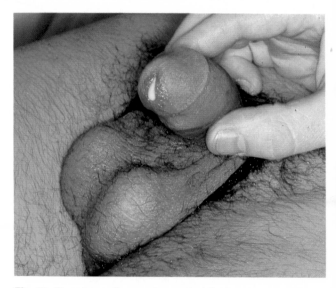

Fig. 17 There is usually a purulent urethral discharge in males with gonococcal urethritis. However, in some cases it may not be so obvious, particularly if the patient has recently voided urine, and in a few cases no discharge is visible at all.

13

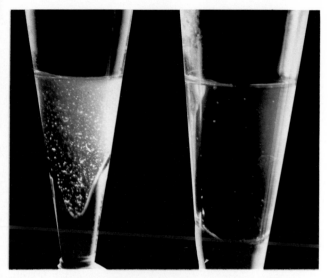

Fig. 18 Uncomplicated urethral gonorrhoea, and indeed, non-specific urethritis, are usually confined to the anterior urethra. In this event the two-glass test will show debris (flakes and threads) in the first glass and clear urine in the second glass. Where a posterior urethritis exists, debris will be found in both glasses and, although a coarse test, it is a rough indicator of the extent of an infection.

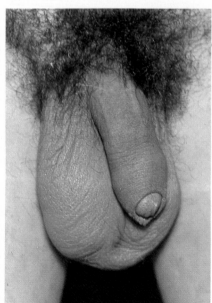

Fig. 19 Where the infection has spread to the posterior urethra, complications such as prostatitis and epididymitis are more likely. In this patient with epididymitis there is painful scrotal swelling on the right due to epididymal thickening and a degree of sympathetic hydrocele formation.

14

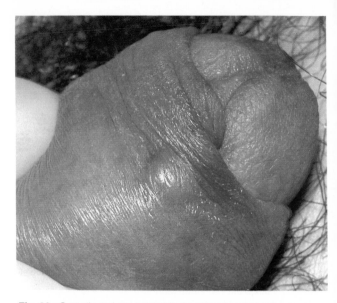

Fig. 20 Complicated gonorrhoea in developed countries is now rare, but local glandular structures such as Tyson's glands, as in this case, can sometimes be inflamed.

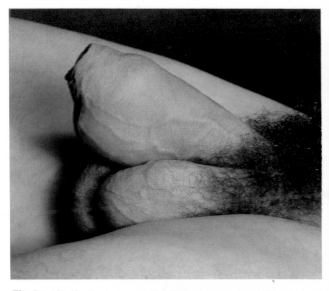

Fig. 21 Littré's glands are usually infected in gonorrhoea. If the ducts of a number of glands become blocked, a periurethral abscess may form although this is now a rare complication.

15

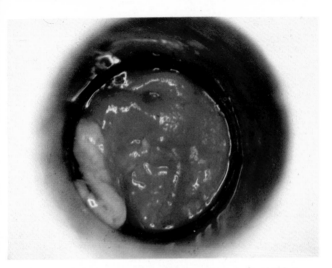

Fig. 22 Gonorrhoea may also infect the rectum. It may reach this site as a result of anal intercourse. In severe cases there can be considerable discomfort, an anal discharge, pain and the passage of bloody mucus on defaecation. Patients are often asymptomatic, especially women, as in this case, where the infection reaches the rectum by spread from the vagina across the perineum.

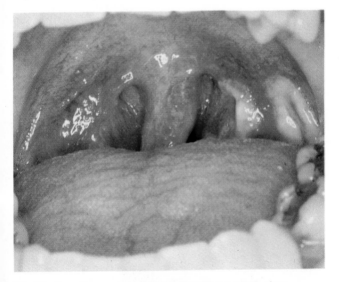

Fig. 23 Sometimes a gonococcal pharyngitis can occur, often asymptomatically, resulting from orogenital sexual contact. There are no special features at this site and the infection is thought by some to be eradicated spontaneously if treatment is not exhibited.

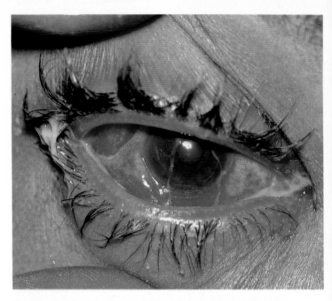

Fig. 24 Accidental autoinoculation of infected material from the genital area to the eye can result in a marked conjunctivitis. Prompt treatment is advisable in order to prevent damage to the cornea.

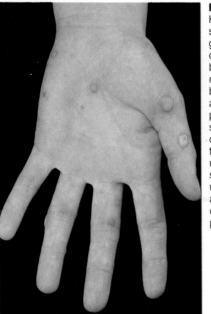

Fig. 25
Haematogenous spread of the gonococcus can occur. The initial bacteraemic phase may be characterised by fever, skin lesions and a migratory polyarthralgia. The skin lesions are clinically similar to those found in meningococcal septicaemia. They may occur almost anywhere but are most commonly found at the peripheries of limbs.

17

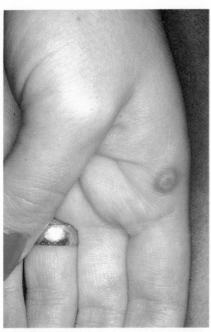

Fig. 26 The lesions start as erythematous papules and often become pustular and haemorrhagic with necrotic centres. They may heal spontaneously and new lesions can occur in an adjacent area. Patients with this complication usually have had a previously asymptomatic gonococcal infection and are therefore often women. It is difficult to identify gonococci from these skin lesions by conventional means.

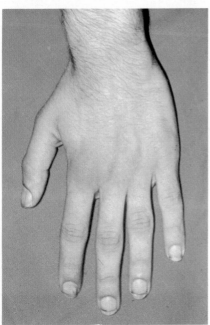

Fig. 27 The bacteraemic phase may resolve spontaneously or the infection may localise in one or more joints producing a septic arthritis. If antibiotics are exhibited rapidly, the arthritis will resolve completely. Other forms of disseminated infection, such as perihepatitis, endocarditis and meningitis are very rare.

18

Vaginal discharge

Most women notice a degree of vaginal secretion sufficient to stain the underwear at the end of the day. The amount of this secretion will vary from person to person and there is no doubt that some women produce more normally constituted vaginal secretion than others. There may also be physiological variation in the amount of secretion, as in pregnancy when it tends to be increased, during sexual arousal, and there can be a menstrual cyclical variation.

Aetiology of increased vaginal secretion

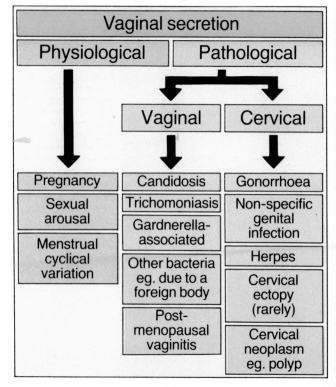

Vaginal secretion		
Physiological	Pathological	
	Vaginal	Cervical
Pregnancy	Candidosis	Gonorrhoea
Sexual arousal	Trichomoniasis	Non-specific genital infection
Menstrual cyclical variation	Gardnerella-associated	Herpes
	Other bacteria eg. due to a foreign body	Cervical ectopy (rarely)
	Post-menopausal vaginitis	Cervical neoplasm eg. polyp

The complaint of discharge is thus a very subjective one as different women will regard varying amounts of secretion as abnormal or excessive. Pathological discharge, however, emanates from either the vagina itself or from the cervix. Trichomoniasis is probably the commonest cause of vaginal discharge worldwide, although in the Western World candidal infection is more common. Both these infections are often associated with vulval pruritis and between them they account for the majority of cases of discharge. However, in recent years, *Gardnerella vaginalis* associated discharge is being diagnosed more frequently. Bacterial vaginitis is rare in healthy adults although it can occur in prepubertal girls. In adults it is most commonly associated with a foreign body such as a retained tampon. Finally, vaginal discharge can be associated with oestrogen deprivation in post-menopausal women.

Cervical infections can often be accompanied by a vaginal discharge but are virtually never associated with pruritis. Many bacteria can produce a cervicitis but *Neisseria gonorrhoeae* and non-specific genital infection, often due to *Chlamydia trachomatis*, are relatively common causes. Ascending infection from the cervix may result in salpingitis, one of the more common complications of gonococcal and chlamydial infections in women. While shedding of the Herpes hominis virus from the cervix is not always associated with visible signs, where lesions are present a profuse discharge may be found. Cervical ectopy on its own does not produce a significant discharge, but if very extensive or secondarily infected it may. A cervical polyp may produce a mucoid discharge and the presence of an intrauterine contraceptive device (IUCD) can be accompanied by an excessive secretion. Cervical neoplasms, although not often seen in young women, may cause vaginal discharge, possibly blood-stained and lesions higher up in the genital tract may also produce a blood-stained discharge.

Candidosis

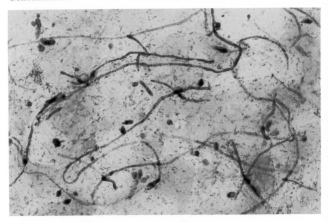

Fig. 28 Vaginal candidosis (thrush) is caused by fungi of the genus *Candida,* the commonest one being *Candida albicans*. This species is characterised by its ability to produce pseudohyphae (chains of elongated yeast cells) and the inability to develop ascospores. Symptoms and signs are unreliable for diagnosis and the microscopic detection of pseudohyphae in Gram-stained smears of discharge is useful. Diagnosis is confirmed by isolation of *Candida* in culture.

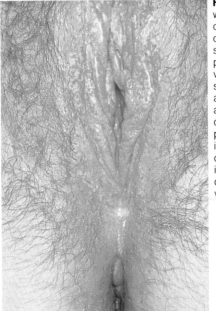

Fig. 29 In patients with vaginal candidosis, pruritis is often the cardinal symptom. Many patients experience vulvo-vaginal soreness, particularly at sexual intercourse, and associated dysuria caused by periurethral inflammation may occur. This picture illustrates a typical case of candidal vulvo-vaginitis.

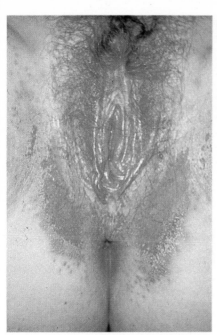

Fig. 30 Sometimes primary cutaneous candidosis of the vulva can occur, unrelated to vaginitis, again the main symptom being pruritis.

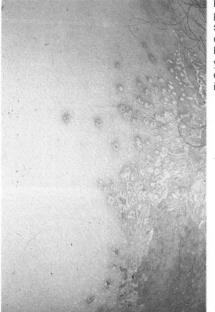

Fig. 31 A close-up of part of the last picture shows the characteristic satellite lesions indicative of a yeast rather than dermatophyte infection.

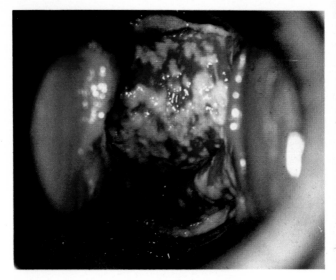

Fig. 32 Vaginal discharge is not invariably associated with vulvo-vaginal candidosis. When present, the discharge is classically thick, lumpy, white and adherent, as in this case, and may have a pungent odour. However, it can be white or creamy and watery. Women who are pregnant, debilitated, immunocompromised or who are taking antibiotics are more likely to develop symptoms.

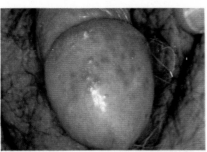

Fig. 33 Although not primarily a sexually transmitted disease, candidal balanitis can sometimes occur; it is usually associated with vaginal candidosis in the sexual partner.

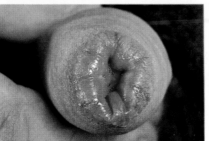

Fig. 34 Posthitis, or inflammation of the prepuce, may also occur. In this case oedema of the prepuce with fissuring has occurred due to hypersensitivity to *Candida*. Candidal urethritis is rare.

23

Trichomoniasis

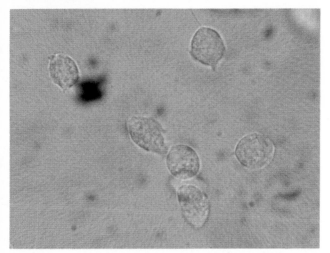

Fig. 35 Trichomonal vaginitis is caused by the flagellate protozoan *Trichomonas vaginalis.* It is easily visualised by taking some discharge from the posterior fornix, placing it on a drop of saline on a slide, covering it with a cover slip and microscopy, using dark ground or reduced transmitted illumination, will reveal a mobile flagellate organism.

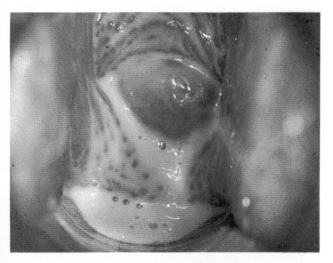

Fig. 36 The infestation may be asymptomatic or may produce acute changes with a profuse, frothy, greenish-yellow discharge exuding from the inflamed vaginal wall. There is often an odour and usually vulval pruritis associated with the condition.

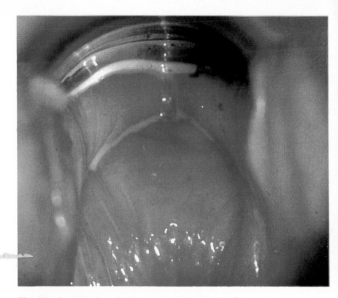

Fig. 37 A marked vaginitis is present in about half the cases.

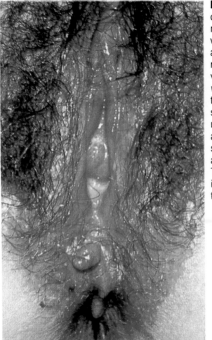

Fig. 38 Sometimes considerable vulvitis may occur associated with prutitis, soreness and dyspareunia. It is not as common as vaginitis. *Trichomonas vaginalis* is usually transmitted by the sexual route. Most male consorts are asymptomatic but some have symptoms and signs of urethritis. They should be investigated and treated.

Gardnerella-associated discharge

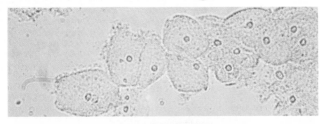

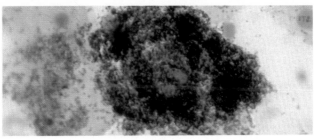

Fig. 39 *Gardnerella vaginalis* is a short Gram-negative coccobacillus. It is found in anaerobic vaginosis. On wet preparation of vaginal secretion it is associated with 'Clue cells'. These are epithelial cells with a granular appearance and with bacteria blurring the epithelial cell margins. They can also be seen on a Gram-stained preparation.

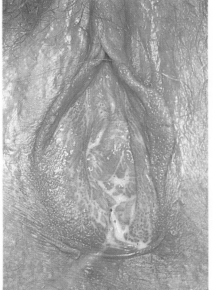

Fig. 40 On inspection of the vestibule, a malodorous grey vaginal discharge may be visible. There is no vulvitis nor pruritis. The odour is often most noticeable after sexual intercourse.

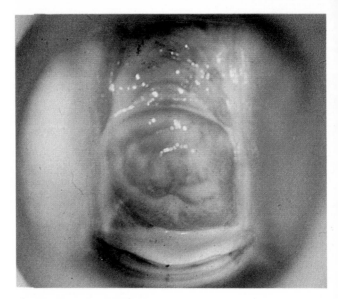

Fig. 41 The grey-white discharge is usually homogenous and when mixed with potassium hydroxide an ammoniacal odour is released. The vaginal pH is greater than 5.0. It is not established that this type of infection is always sexually transmitted.

Non-specific cervicitis

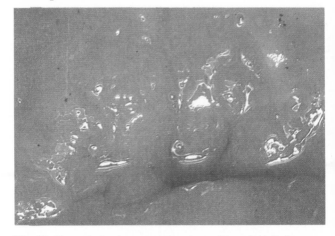

Fig. 42 The majority of women with non-specific genital infection (NSGI) are asymptomatic. Yellow vaginal discharge resulting from pus production by an infected cervix is the commonest symptom, when any exist. In long-standing infection with *Chlamydia trachomatis*, follicles may be visible on the cervix as in this case.

27

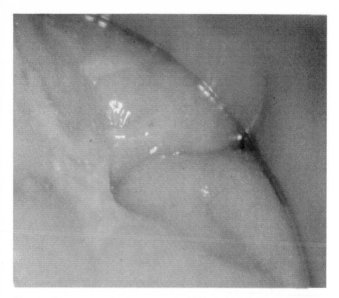

Fig. 43 Chlamydial infection can spread from the cervix to the rectum, or can be introduced there by means of anal intercourse, although it is not commonly transmitted by homosexual men. The infection is usually asymptomatic but marked pus production can be seen on proctoscopy.

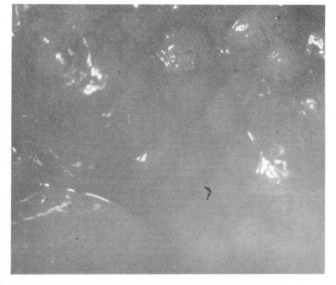

Fig. 44 Sometimes, in cases of long-standing infection, a follicular or 'cobblestone' appearance may be visible in the rectum.

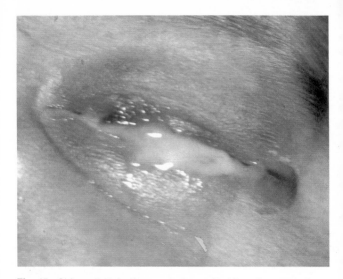

Fig. 45 Chlamydial infection may be transmitted from the maternal cervix to the baby's conjunctival sac during parturition. *Chlamydia trachomatis* is now probably the commonest cause of ophthalmia neonatorum in Europe and North America. The incubation period is usually about 6 days.

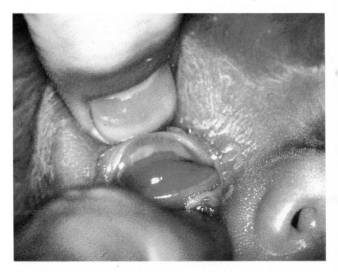

Fig. 46 Considerable conjunctival mucoidal oedema may occur with chlamydial infection. Proper treatment consists of tetracycline eye ointment instillations. Systemic erythromycin should be added and it should also prevent the subsequent development of a chlamydial pneumonia, 5-8 weeks later.

29

Gonococcal cervicitis

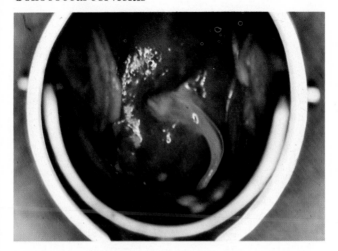

Fig. 47 The majority of women with uncomplicated gonorrhoea have few noticeable symptoms. When present, the commonest one is a yellow, often malodorous but non-pruritic vaginal discharge. This emanates from a gonococcal cervicitis.

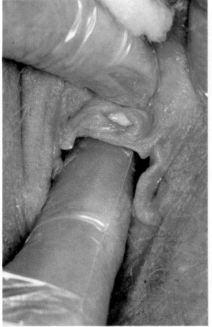

Fig. 48 Sometimes, where urethritis is present, it may be possible to express pus from the urethral orifice. Dysuria and urinary frequency may be noticed in these cases.

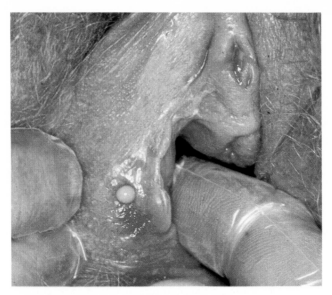

Fig. 49 While gonorrhoea is uncomplicated at the majority of sites, it may be a complication which first draws attention to the infection. Here gonococcal pus may be seen extending from a Bartholin's duct.

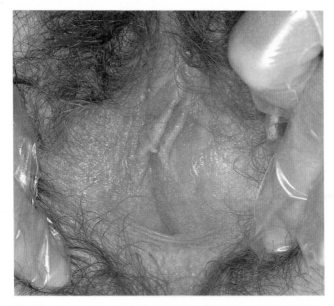

Fig. 50 Where a Bartholin's duct becomes blocked, an abscess of the duct may result producing a painful vulval swelling.

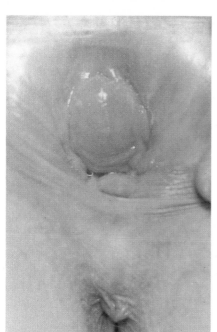

Fig. 51 A painful swelling due to a periurethral abscess can also occur occasionally.

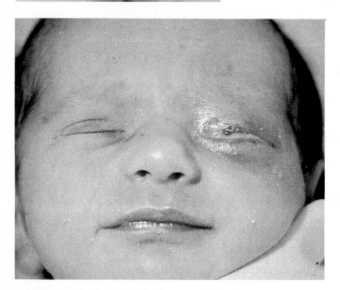

Fig. 52 As with chlamydial infection, gonorrhoea may cause ophthalmia neonatorum. Signs usually appear within 2-5 days of delivery and the inflammation and resultant oedema is more marked than with a chlamydial infection.

Genital ulceration

The presence of genital ulcers or sores is another common reason for presentation at a STD clinic. These lesions may generate great anxiety and patients may suspect quite innocent lesions of being sexually acquired.

The commonest cause of genital ulceration in the Western World is genital herpes, which has increased dramatically in incidence in North America and Europe in recent years. Syphilis, although not seen as frequently as in years gone by, is still a significant infection and can produce ulceration in the primary stage as a chancre, in the secondary stage as mucous patches, and in the tertiary stage as gummatous ulcers. Tertiary syphilis is, however, rare nowadays. In tropical countries the trio of chancroid, lymphogranuloma venereum and granuloma inguinale may be seen, and in many areas such as Africa and South East Asia, chancroid is probably the commonest cause of ulceration. All of these conditions can be associated with inguinal lymphadenopathy.

It is important to bear in mind simple pyogenic lesions which can ulcerate and are not uncommon in the hairy parts of the genital area. Scabies usually produces itching, and scratching may result in ulceration and secondary infection. Trauma, usually induced by sexual activity, may produce fissuring of the skin particularly in the coronal sulcus in men and in the fourchette area in women. This tends to be more common when skin conditions such as seborrhoeic eczema are present. Severe balanitis due to a variety of causes may result in erosion of the glans penis, for example in severe candidosis and in Reiter's disease. Drug eruptions and neoplastic disease as well as the rare Behçet's disease can also be responsible for genital ulceration.

In this section only the conditions spread by the sexual route will be represented in the photographs. Examples of scabetic lesions are to be found in the section on infestations, Reiter's disease under non-specific infection in the male and candidal infection under candidosis.

Aetiology of genital ulceration

Infectious lesions
    genital herpes
    syphilis – primary: chancre
                secondary: mucous patches
                tertiary: gumma
    tropical ulcers: chancroid
                lymphogranuloma venereum
                granuloma inguinale
Pyogenic lesions eg. ruptured furuncle
Trauma –
    physical
    chemical
Secondary to infestations eg. scabies
Balanitis –
    severe candidosis
    circinate balanitis in Reiter's disease
    associated with Vincent's organisms
    plasma cell balanitis of Zoon
Drug eruption –
    localised: fixed drug eruption
    generalised: Stevens Johnson syndrome
Neoplastic conditions –
    carcinoma
    premalignant condition: erythroplasia
                of Queyrat
Rarities –
    Behçet's disease
    tuberculous ulceration

Herpes

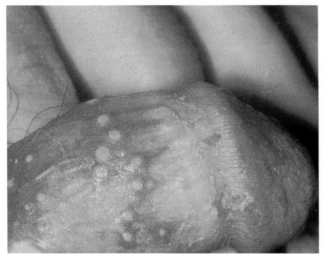

Fig. 53 Some 4-5 days after contact, vesicles will appear in the affected area, in this case on the penis. The lesions are not generally painful at this stage. In recurrent episodes a prodrome such as an ache in the thighs may precede an attack.

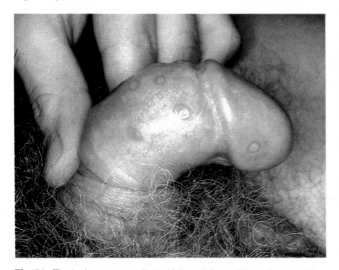

Fig. 54 The lesions are usually multiple and the vesicles subsequently rupture, leaving painful superficial erosions with a characteristic erythematous surround. They are most often found, as here, on the undersurface of the retracted prepuce in the coronal sulcus, although any part of the penis may be affected.

35

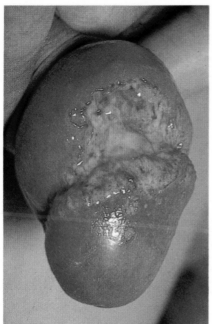

Fig. 55 Sometimes the erosions can become confluent and a more extensive area of ulceration may result. This can become secondarily infected with bacteria and may be extremely painful.

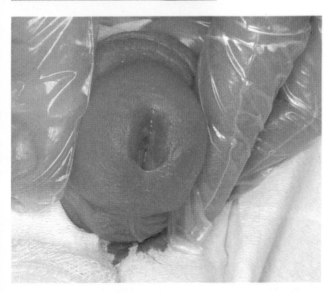

Fig. 56 Herpesvirus infection can affect the urethral meatus and lead to dysuria and urethral discharge, thus mimicking the symptoms of non-specific urethritis. Urinary retention may also occur.

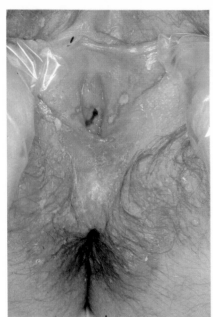

Fig. 57 Vesicles are visible in the perianal area but have ruptured at the fourchette and on the inner surfaces of the labia minora to reveal the characteristic herpetic erosions.

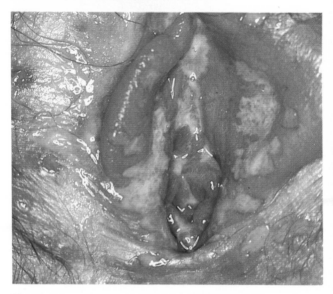

Fig. 58 The lesions here have become almost confluent, they are slightly necrotic in appearance and are associated with a degree of vulval oedema. The degree of pain did not permit speculum examination of this patient.

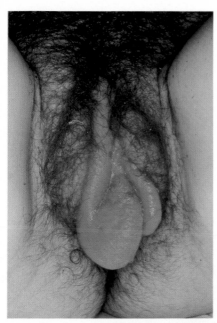

Fig. 59 Herpetic lesions are visible on this oedematous vulva. This generally only occurs in a primary attack and can be associated with retention of urine necessitating suprapubic catheterisation.

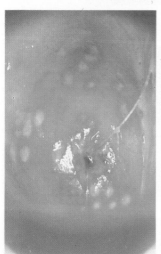

Fig. 60 The cervix can shed herpesvirus without any external signs. Here, vesicles and erosions are visible.

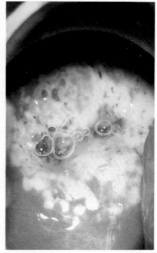

Fig. 61 A more extensive degree of ulceration can occur, with a necrotic appearance and profuse mucus secretion. Virus culture to confirm the diagnosis would be advisable in this case.

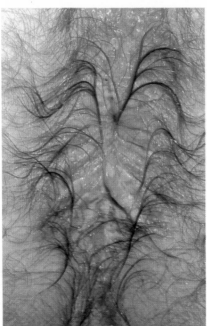

Fig. 62 Perianal herpes can occur in both sexes, but is now seen quite commonly in male homosexuals, as in this case. The degree of discomfort can make defaecation difficult and an herpetic proctitis can also exist in some cases. Urinary retention is also sometimes associated with infection at this site.

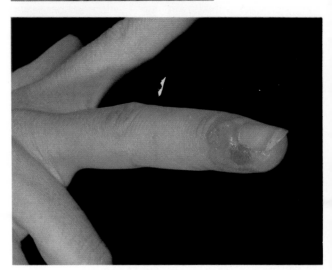

Fig. 63 An herpetic whitlow can sometimes occur when a finger is contaminated from an infected genital site. Should such a whitlow be present in the puerperium, then particular care is required in handling the newborn baby which could be at risk of acquiring a generalised herpes infection.

39

Primary syphilis

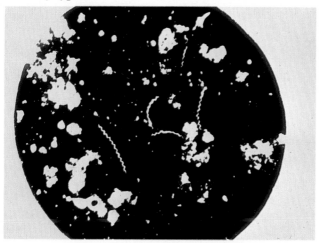

Fig. 64 Syphilis is caused by *Treponema pallidum*. The organism can be visualised by dark ground microscopic examination of scrapings taken from the primary lesion of syphilis – a chancre, or from mucous lesions and condylomata lata in the secondary stage. The organisms are spiral, motile and can be seen to angulate and rotate.

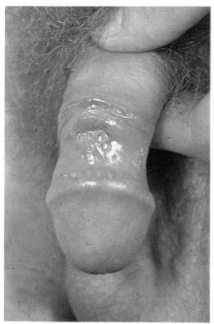

Fig. 65 Primary chancre of the penis. The skin of the coronal sulcus is usually stretched during sexual activity and the treponeme frequently enters at this site. A chancre then appears some time in the following 9-90 days; usually about 3-4 weeks after infection.

40

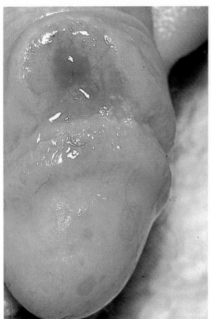

Fig. 66 The chancre begins as a macule which soon becomes papular and is then eroded leaving an ulcer. The lesion may be indurated with raised edges and is hard or firm to palpation. There may be oedema of adjacent tissues.

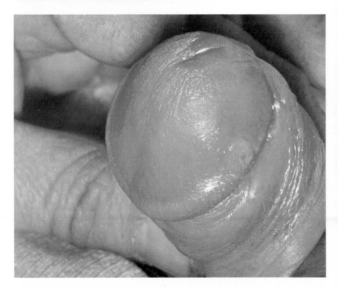

Fig. 67 A chancre can appear at any site on the penis, here on the glans. As the lesions are usually painless and often small, in the uncircumcised man they can pass unnoticed until they heal spontaneously over 4-8 weeks.

41

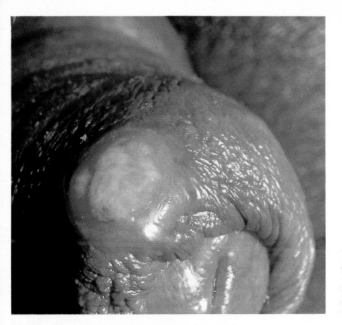

Fig. 68 Primary chancre of the prepuce of the penis.

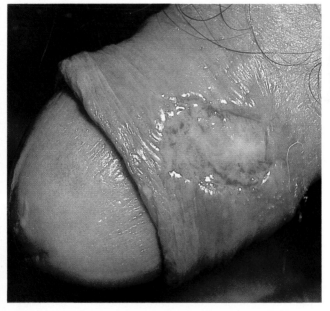

Fig. 69 Chancre of the retracted prepuce.

42

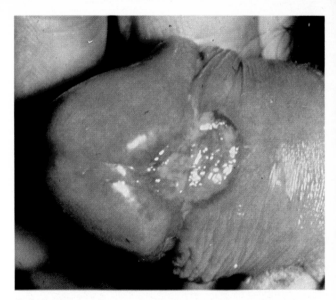

Fig. 70 The fraenum of the penis is a relatively common site for a primary chancre. While chancres usually heal without scarring, the fraenum can sometimes be destroyed by the process.

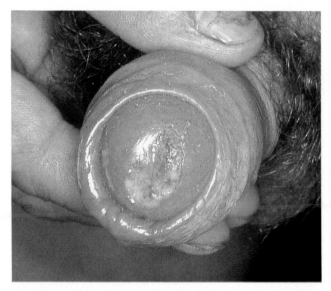

Fig. 71 A chancre can arise at the urethral meatus. Although in this case it is quite obvious, separation of the meatal edges may be required to demonstrate the lesion.

43

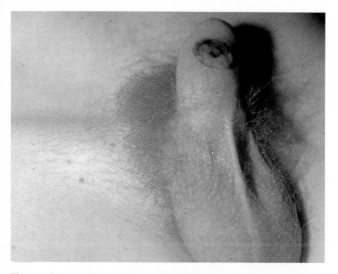

Fig. 72 Primary chancre of the penis with inguinal lymphadenopathy. The inguinal glands begin to enlarge soon after the appearance of the chancre. The glands are characteristically discrete, rubbery, mobile and non-tender. Glandular enlargement is found in the majority of cases and resolution can take several months.

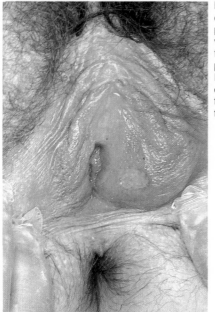

Fig. 73 The characteristics of a primary chancre of the vulva are the same as for a chancre on the penis, or elsewhere. Lesions are most commonly found on the inner aspects of the labia minora.

44

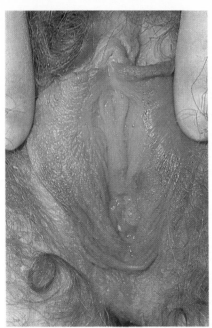

Fig. 74 As vulval chancres are often small, painless and sometimes at sites not usually noticeable to the patient, it is possible for the patient to pass through the primary stage of syphilis without being aware of the infection.

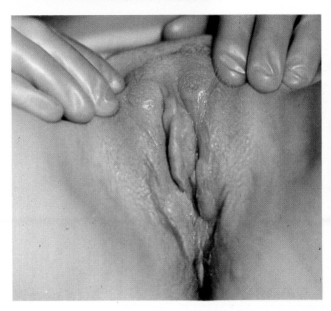

Fig. 75 This patient has two so-called 'kissing chancres' on the labia majora.

45

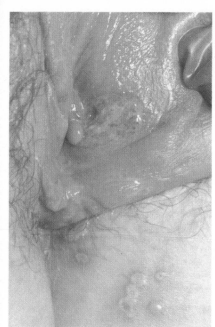

Fig. 76 This patient has a typical primary chancre of the vulva but in addition has visible vesicular and erosive lesions of genital herpes, a reminder that more than one STD can exist in any patient.

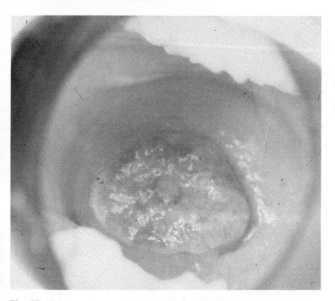

Fig. 77 Primary chancre of the cervix. A patient has no means of knowing when a chancre appears on the cervix and so will probably infect a sexual partner.

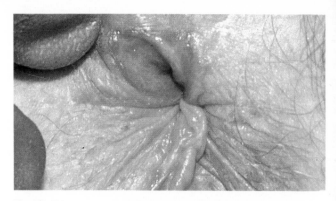

Fig. 78 Primary chancre of the anus. An individual chancre can appear at the anal margin and can resemble a fissure, although it is not usually painful. Eversion of the anal edges may be necessary to reveal the lesions. Frequently the patient may not notice a primary lesion at this site and the first appreciable sign of syphilis may be when the secondary manifestations appear. The anus should always be inspected in patients being examined for sexually transmitted diseases, especially homosexual males or those practising anal intercourse.

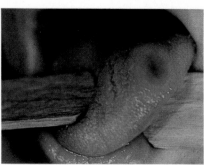

Fig. 79 Primary chancre of the tongue. Chancres are not always confined to genital sites. Orogenital sexual contact is common and so manifestations of primary syphilis may appear in the mouth.

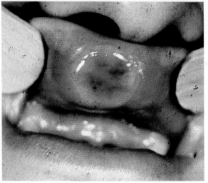

Fig. 80 Primary chancre of the lip.

47

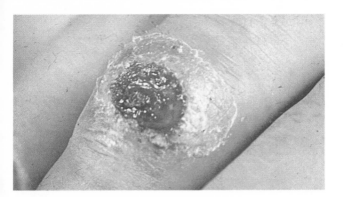

Fig. 81 Chancres can appear on the fingers as a result of digital contact with the genital area.

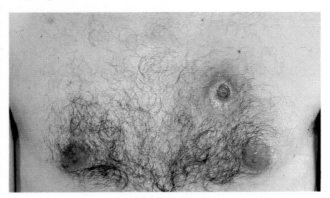

Fig. 82 Primary chancre of the chest wall. This patient was bitten by his girlfriend and treponemes were presumably introduced in this way.

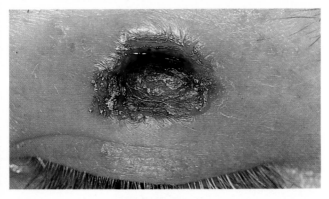

Fig. 83 Primary chancre of the eyelid.

Secondary syphilis

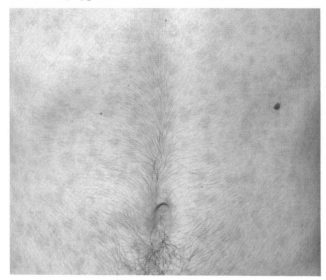

Fig. 84 The rash of secondary syphilis, a syphilide, occurs in about three-quarters of the patients in this stage of the disease. It usually arises about 6-8 weeks after the onset of the primary stage. (The chancre may still be present in about one-third of patients at the onset of the secondary stage). The rash begins in the macular stage as here and is commonly first seen at the costal margins.

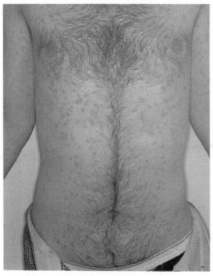

Fig. 85 The rash can be quite diffuse and is rarely seen in only one stage. Its most frequent presentation is in the maculopapular stage (usually being polymorphic).

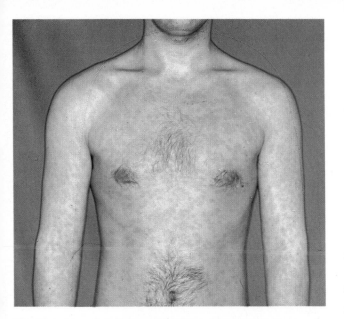

Fig. 86 In this patient, the maculopapular rash is seen on the trunk and also on the arms. The flexor surfaces of the forearms are frequently affected sites.

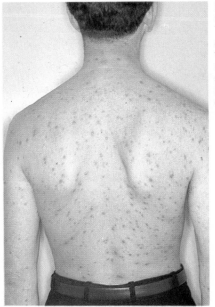

Fig. 87 A papular syphilide is also seen. The rash is rarely itchy and may persist for weeks or months if untreated. It is always symmetrical. Cellular infiltration has occurred at this stage.

50

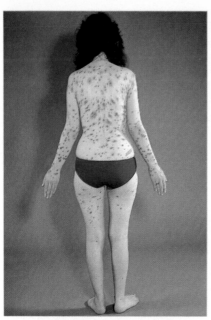

Fig. 88 A papular rash can be quite marked and indolent, but generally heals without any scarring.

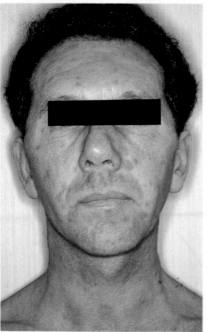

Fig. 89 This patient has a papular rash of the face, although the face is not as often affected as lower parts of the body.

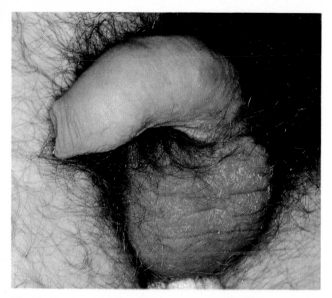

Fig. 90 Papules may be seen on the penis, where they must be differentiated from other conditions such as scabies and furunculosis.

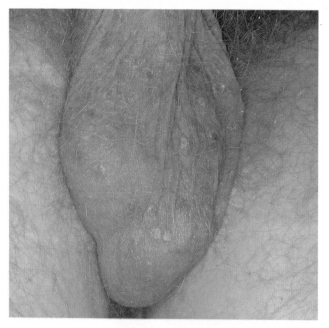

Fig. 91 The scrotum can also be involved in the papular stage.

52

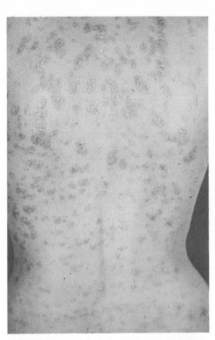

Fig. 92 Sometimes the rash can become scaly or psoriasiform: the so-called papulo-squamous syphilide.

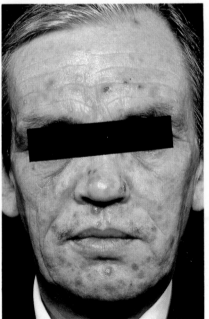

Fig. 93 Papular lesions can occasionally undergo central necrosis leading to the papulo-pustular or papulo-necrotic stage. Healing at this stage may result in residual scarring.

53

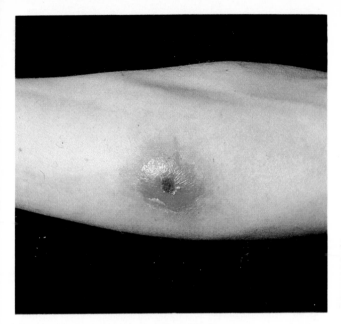

Fig. 94 A large papulonecrotic lesion of the forearm.

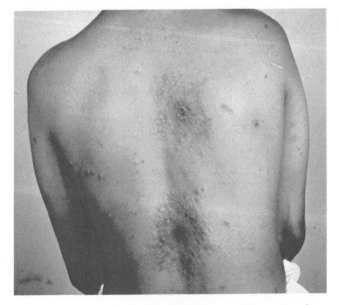

Fig. 95 Occasionally a large central lesion is seen with a number of surrounding satellite lesions – so-called corymbose syphilide.

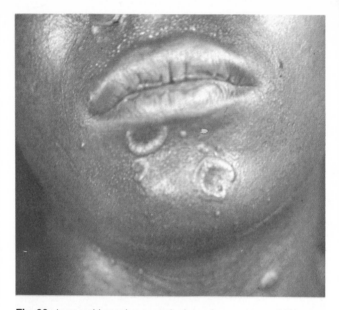

Fig. 96 In negroid people an annular form of secondary syphilide may be seen.

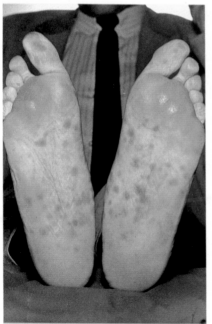

Fig. 97 In the papular stage of the rash, lesions may appear on the palms of the hands and the soles of the feet. At these sites they are virtually pathognomonic of secondary syphilis. In this patient, typical lesions are seen on the soles.

55

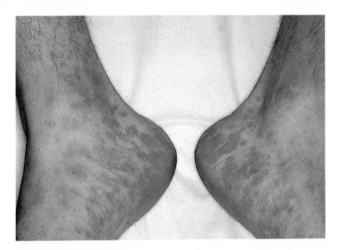

Fig. 98 Sometimes the soles themselves may not be so obviously affected and lesions may be most easily seen on the medial aspects of the foot arches, below the medial malleoli.

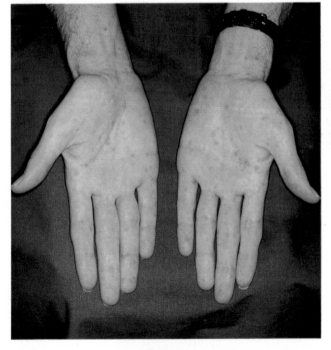

Fig. 99 When the soles are affected there are often lesions on the palms as well. In this patient palmar syphilide is easily seen.

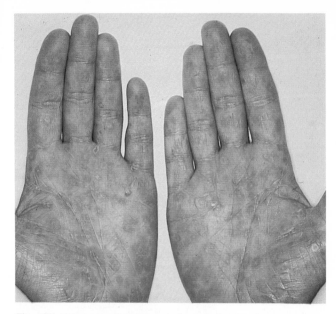

Fig. 100 Palmar manifestations can be quite florid, and squamous change may be seen, although not particularly so in this case.

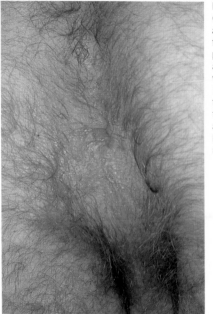

Fig. 101
Condylomata lata appear as raised fleshy wart-like papules in the hotter areas of the body where friction occurs. In the papular stage they occur mainly in the perianal and vulval areas. In this case the lesion is at the anal margin.

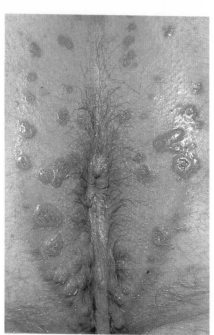

Fig. 102
Condylomata lata
lesions are usually
multiple.

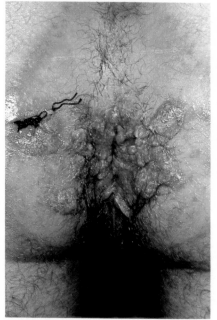

Fig. 103 Sometimes
condylomata can
become very fleshy in
appearance. They
exude serum which is
teeming with
Treponema pallidum.
They are thus highly
infectious lesions.

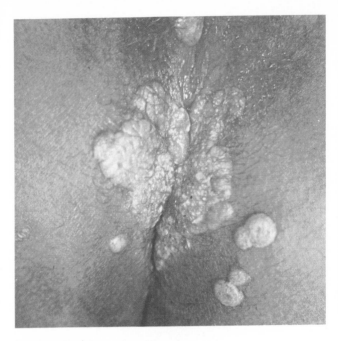

Fig. 104 Condylomata lata of the vulva.

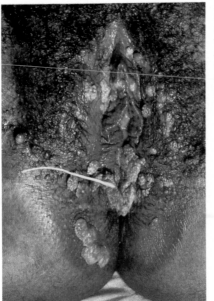

Fig. 105
Condylomata lata
must be differentiated
from condylomata
accuminata.
Occasionally the two
can coexist, as in this
patient

59

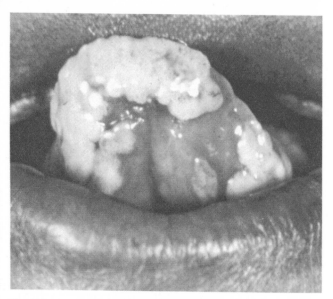

Fig. 106 Non-genital sites can also be affected with condylomata lata, as here on the tongue. They are also seen in the groin, on the thigh, at the angle of the mouth, in the axilla, or under a pendulous breast. In addition the penis and scrotum can be affected.

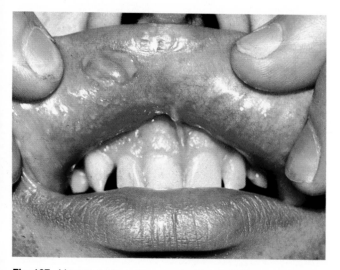

Fig. 107 Mucous patch on the upper lip. Mucous lesions occur at the same time as the cutaneous manifestations of secondary syphilis. They are found most commonly on the buccal mucosa but also on the pharynx and larynx.

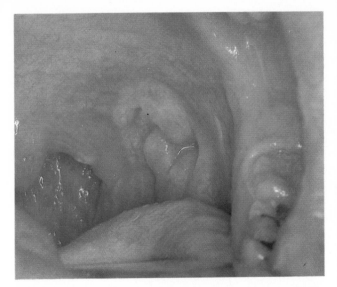

Fig. 108 Mucous lesions of the mouth are usually painless superficial erosions. Sometimes small lesions may coalesce to produce a lesion with a serpiginous outline ('snail-trail ulcer'). Mucous lesions are highly infectious.

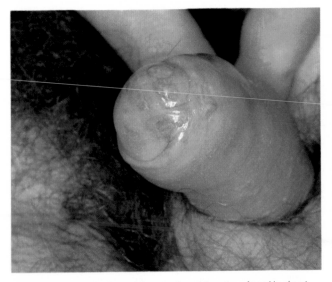

Fig. 109 Mucous lesions of the mouth and throat are found in about one-third of cases of secondary syphilis. They are also seen in the genital area; in the male they may be found beneath the prepuce and on the glans penis, as in this patient.

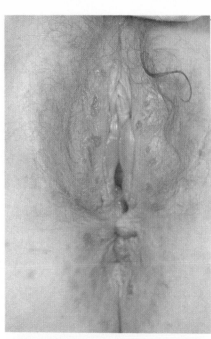

Fig. 110 In women, the lesions can be seen on the vulva, as here, but also rarely on the vaginal wall and cervix.

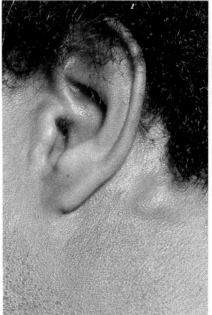

Fig. 111 In secondary syphilis about half the patients have a degree of generalised lymphadenopathy. This patient has a visible enlarged cervical node.

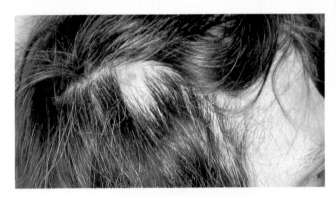

Fig. 112 Alopecia. In the papular stage of secondary syphilis, papules can appear on the scalp and there can be a patchy hair loss in the area, as in this patient. Whether treated or not, the hair will grow again.

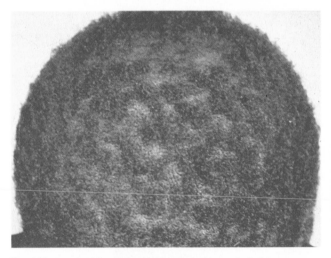

Fig. 113 In negroid people with short hair, this patchy hair loss may take on a characteristic appearance, the so-called 'moth-eaten' scalp.

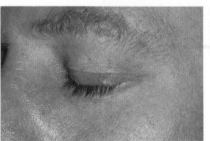

Fig. 114 Syphilitic alopecia – hair has been lost at the lateral part of the eyebrow.

Late forms of syphilis

After the early infectious stages of syphilis, the untreated sufferer passes into the latent stage of the disease. Many will subsequently die from causes totally unrelated to their treponemal infection. However some may develop tertiary syphilis, usually between 3 and 12 years after the primary infection. The cardiovascular and central nervous systems are invaded by the treponeme in the secondary stage of syphilis, but it is only many years later that symptoms and signs of disease in these systems may manifest themselves. The late forms of syphilis are rarely seen in the developed world today.

TERTIARY OR GUMMATOUS SYPHILIS

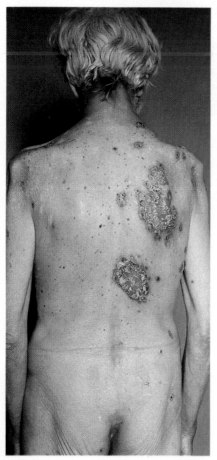

Fig. 115 The lesion of tertiary syphilis – the gumma, can affect almost any structure in the body, but skin and bone are among the most commonly affected sites. Here the back is involved with superficial, painless, dull red lesions, which can actually occur on any part of the skin surface – nodular cutaneous syphilide.

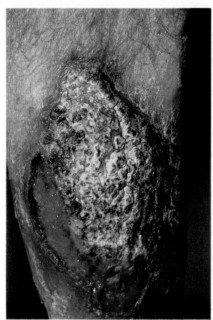

Fig. 116 The lesions are often multiple and can be psoriasiform or scaly. The dependent lymph nodes are not enlarged. Healing can occur spontaneously, but often, when it does, another lesion may develop in an adjacent area. There may be 'tissue-paper' scars at the site of a healed lesion.

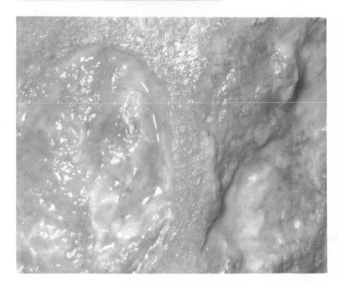

Fig. 117 Subcutaneous tissues may be affected too. Here are two punched-out ulcers revealing the destructive ability of the gummatous process. The yellowish-white slough at the bases of the lesions is often known as the 'wash-leather slough'. There is residual tissue loss in these cases when healing occurs.

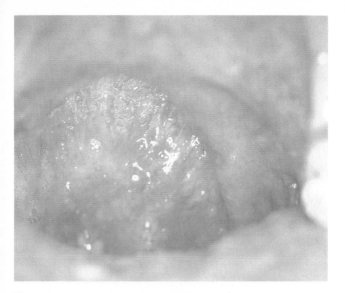

Fig. 118 Mucous surfaces can be affected by the gummatous process; mucous lesions are often the most destructive and in this patient the uvula was completely destroyed.

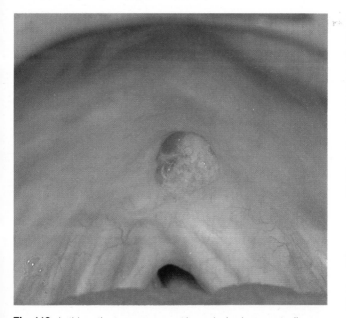

Fig. 119 In this patient a mucous membrane lesion has eventually eroded through the hard palate.

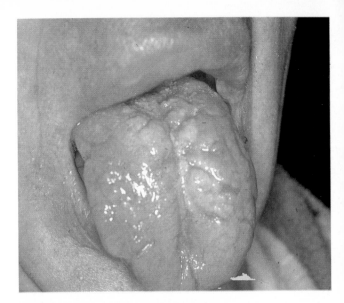

Fig. 120 Diffuse gummatous infiltration of the tongue may occur and result in 'chronic superficial glossitis'. The tongue eventually appears lobulated, has loss of papillae and often develops areas of leukoplakia.

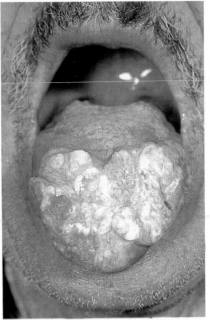

Fig. 121 Diffuse gummatous infiltration can sometimes result in malignant change. In this case the lobulation of the tongue is obvious, as is leukoplakia and a squamous carcinoma.

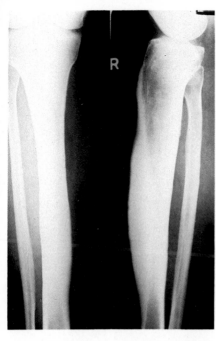

Fig. 122 Any bone can be affected by gummatous lesions, however the skull bones and the tibiae are most commonly affected, and a deep-seated boring pain may be associated with the lesions. Although the lesions can be destructive, the process usually results in new bone formation in the cortical area so that bones may be thickened irregularly. This can be obvious in the anterior third of the tibia, as in this case, where the apparent bowing earns the name 'sabre tibia'. Bone is actually strengthened in these circumstances.

CARDIOVASCULAR SYPHILIS

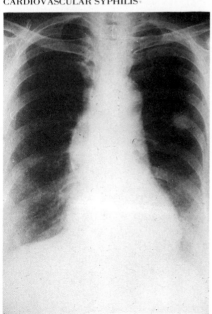

Fig. 123 The aorta is the most commonly affected vessel and the pathological changes there can lead to aortic dilatation with aneurysm and to aortic regurgitation. In this patient aneurysm of the ascending aorta is seen (the commonest site) and the linear calcification in that area is virtually pathognomonic of the disease.

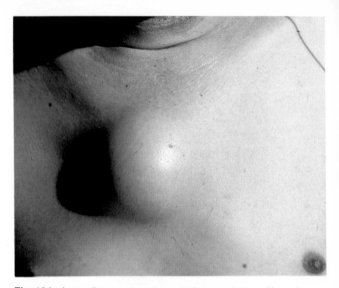

Fig. 124 Ascending aneurysms can project anteriorly and here the aneurysm is seen to have eroded the sternum. Death will occur upon rupture of the vessel.

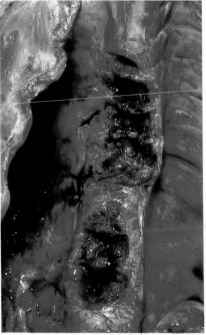

Fig. 125 Aneurysms can also project posteriorly and erode the vertebrae, as in this case. Damage to the spine can occur.

69

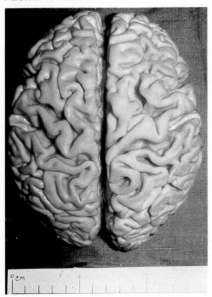

Fig. 126 With general paralysis of the insane (GPI) there is progressive degeneration of the parenchyma of the brain, producing mental and physical deterioration and eventually complete dementia and paralysis, with incontinence. Post mortem inspection of the brain shows it to be shrunken, with widened sulci and small convolutions.

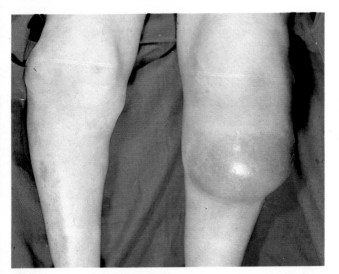

Fig. 127 With parenchymatous degeneration of the posterior columns of the spinal cord in tabes dorsalis, deep sensory loss occurs. As a result, trophic changes can take place, mainly in the weight-bearing joints (Charcot's arthropathy). The knees are commonly affected as in this case where the joints are totally disrupted, and painless. An effusion also exists in the left knee.

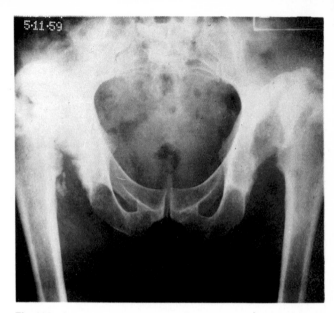

Fig. 128 Charcot's arthropathy may also occur in the hip joints, as in this case, in the lower spine and very occasionally in the upper limbs.

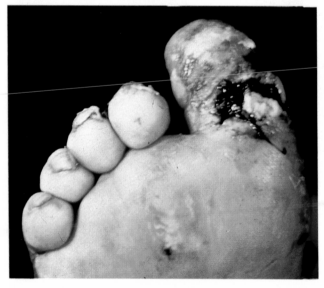

Fig. 129 Trophic changes may also occur on the sole of the foot, the so-called 'perforating ulcer'. New cases of advanced tabes dorsalis are rarely seen in the developed world nowadays.

Congenital syphilis

The term congenital syphilis is a misnomer as it is not a genetically transmitted disease but rather an intrauterine infection, the treponeme crossing the placental barrier from mother to fetus. The incidence of the disease has fallen dramatically in Western countries but the condition is still seen relatively frequently in some developing countries. The spectrum of disease seen in this condition is large and some examples are shown here.

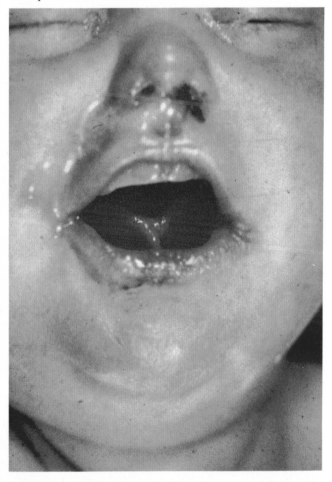

Fig. 130 The nasal mucosa can be affected in early congenital syphilis leading to a profuse nasal discharge which may block the nose, causing the baby to make bubbling sounds when breathing – 'syphilitic snuffles'.

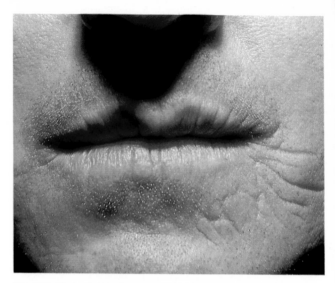

Fig. 131 The rash in early congenital syphilis, when present around the mouth, tends to become fissured as in the previous picture. This can lead to linear scars radiating from the angles of the mouth known as 'rhagades', one of the stigmata of early congenital syphilis.

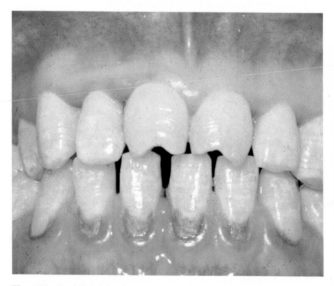

Fig. 132 Syphilitic infection at the time of birth may affect developing tooth buds leading to dental dystrophies. The best known of these is where the central incisors become barrel-shaped and there is notching of the cutting edges – 'Hutchinson's teeth', also a stigma.

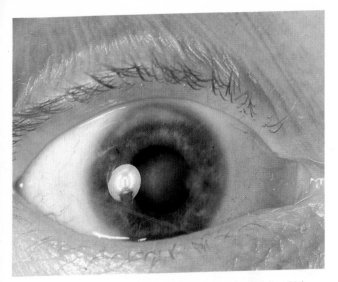

Fig. 133   Another stigma is scarring of the cornea due to interstitial keratitis. It is the commonest late lesion of congenital syphilis, being present in over 25% of cases. A 'ground glass' appearance of the cornea is seen. When present along with Hutchinson's teeth and eighth nerve deafness the patient has 'Hutchinson's triad'.

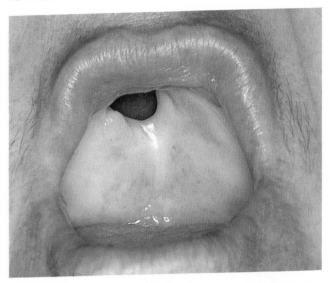

Fig. 134   Gummatous lesions can develop in late congenital syphilis and their destructive nature is illustrated in this patient with a perforated palate.

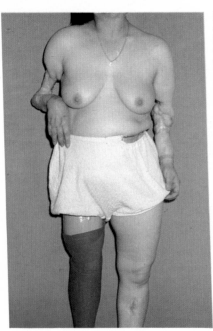

Fig. 135 Gummatous destruction can result in gross scarring and tissue loss. Indeed, in this patient, the right leg was rendered useless and was amputated.

Endemic treponematosis

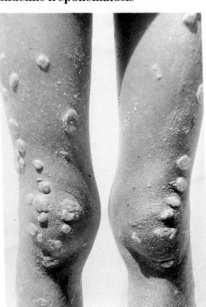

Fig. 136 Secondary yaws. Patients with endemic forms of syphilis, such as yaws, as seen in this child, and pinta and bejel, will also have positive serological tests for syphilis, and this should be borne in mind when dealing with patients from endemic areas.

Chancroid

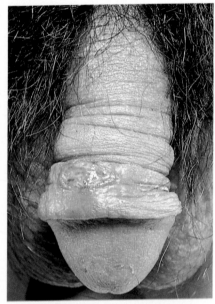

Fig. 137 Chancroid of the penis. After an incubation period of 3–5 days a small vesicopustule may appear, which breaks down into a saucer-shaped ulcer with an erythematous halo. The causative organism is *Haemophilus ducreyi*.

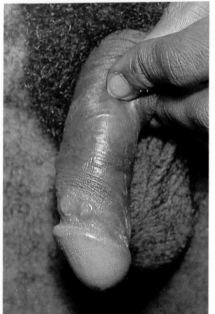

Fig. 138 Autoinoculation can lead to new adjacent lesions appearing. They are tender and painful, but not usually indurated – hence the old name 'soft sore'.

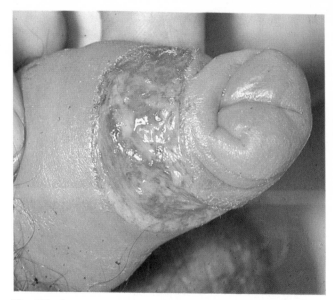

Fig. 139 Sometimes the sores can coalesce to form a large lesion which is usually extremely painful and may be associated with oedema, of the prepuce in this case. There is a tendency to bleed on contact.

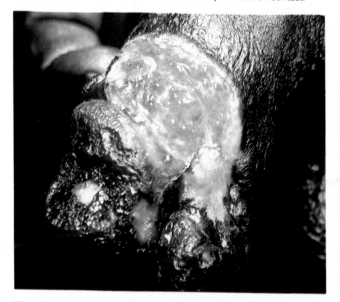

Fig. 140 If the lesions are untreated they can become destructive and penile tissue can be damaged.

77

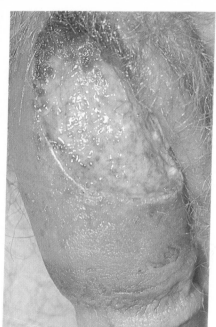

Fig. 141 Any part of the penis can be affected by chancroid, and here the proximal part of the shaft is involved.

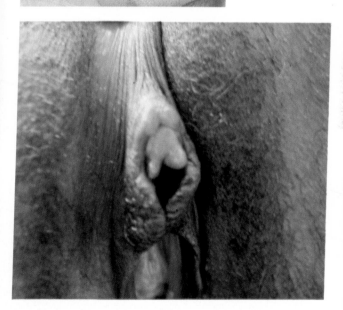

Fig. 142 Lesions are not as commonly seen in the female as in the male, but when present the appearances are similar.

78

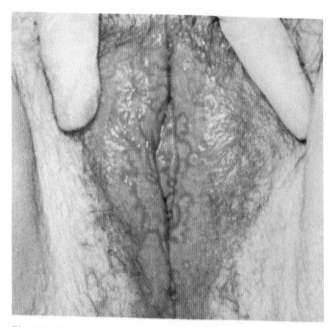

Fig. 143 Chancroid of the vulva can cause extensive ulceration.

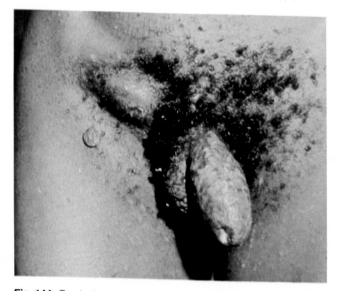

Fig. 144 Tender lymphadenitis, most commonly unilateral, develops in more than 50% of chancroid patients. A bubo can form and may subsequently rupture.

Lymphogranuloma venereum

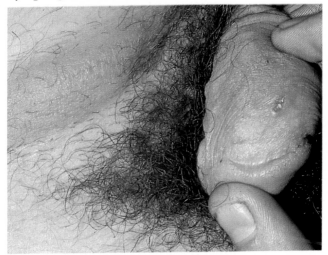

Fig. 145 Between 5-21 days after exposure to infection a small painful, often herpetiform-type erosion may appear on the genitalia. The lesion is transient and not often seen by the doctor. It is the inguinal swelling which usually precipitates the consultation.

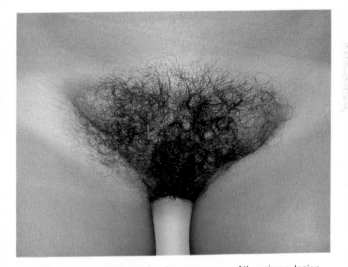

Fig. 146 Some 10-30 days after the appearance of the primary lesion, the inguinal glands become enlarged and tender. The overlying skin can be red and hot and the underlying glands become matted together to form a bubo. The glandular enlargement is bilateral in about two-thirds of cases.

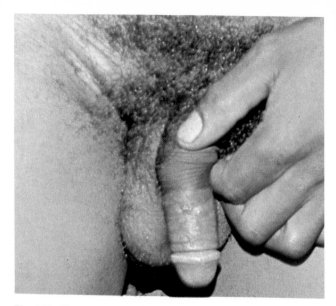

Fig. 147 Simultaneous enlargement of the glands on both sides of the inguinal ligament allows the ligament to bisect the enlargement. This produces the 'groove-sign' which is characteristic of the condition.

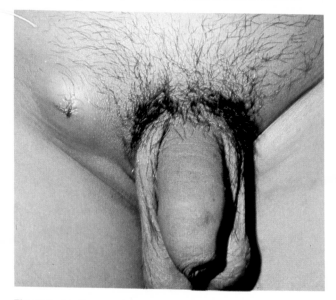

Fig. 148 A bubo can enlarge and become fluctuant. The 'groove-sign' is also seen here.

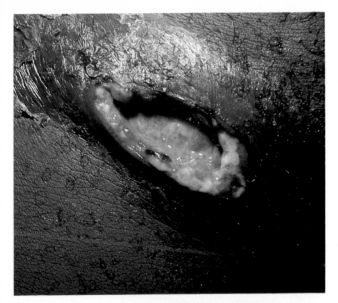

Fig. 149 If the bubo is not aspirated nor treatment instituted the glands may 'break-down' and drain chronically.

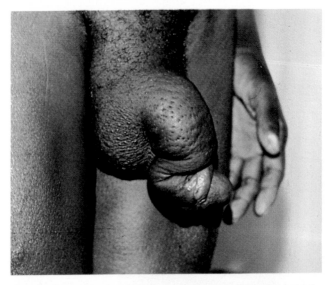

Fig. 150 Where the dorsal lymphatics of the penis are involved, small abscesses may arise in the lymphatic channels leading to tissue destruction and oedema, resulting in elephantiasis or a distortion called 'saxophone penis'.

82

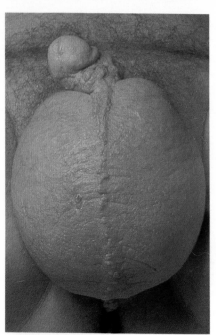

Fig. 151 Scrotal elephantiasis may also occur.

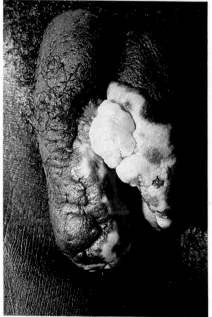

Fig. 152 In females, the lymphatic channels of the vulva may be similarly affected leading to vulval elephantiasis – 'esthiomène'. Sometimes vaginal and rectal strictures or a rectovaginal fistula may occur.

Granuloma inguinale

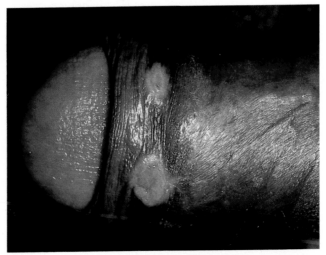

Fig. 153 After a variable incubation period of 1-12 weeks, an ulcer can develop. It is usually painless when secondarily infected and has a scaly appearance. The causative organism is *Calymmatobacterium* (or *Donovania*) *granulomatis*.

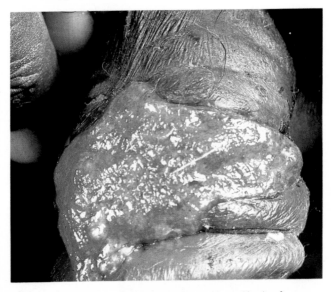

Fig. 154 The lesions can enlarge to leave an ulcer with a beefy granulomatous appearance and a sharply defined, almost rolled edge. There is a tendency to bleed at the touch.

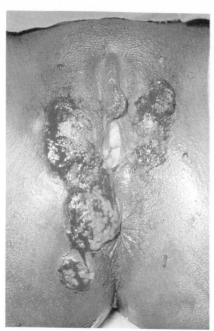

Fig. 155 Granuloma inguinale may spread locally by autoinoculation. Note the raised appearance of the lesions and the tendency to bleeding.

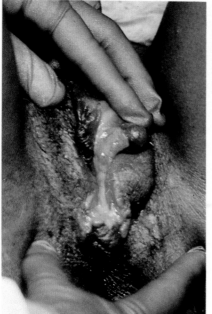

Fig. 156 The perineal and perianal areas can also be affected by granuloma inguinale. The ulceration can, with time, become stationary and areas of spontaneous healing can occur, often with keloid formation.

85

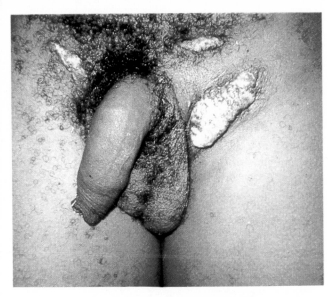

Fig. 157 Inguinal lymphadenopathy is not usual but subcutaneous granulomas can occur, producing swellings in the groin – 'pseudo-buboes'. These may soften into an abscess and burst.

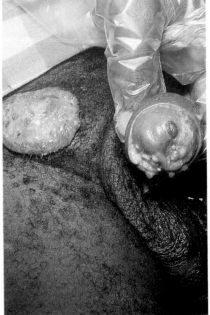

Fig. 158 Both the penis and the groin can be affected by granuloma inguinale.

Genital warts, molluscum contagiosum, infestations and Kaposi's sarcoma

If candidosis is excluded, condylomata accuminata (genital warts) are the third most commonly notified STD in the United Kingdom. The condition is caused by the human wart or papillomavirus. The incubation period is variable, is usually less than three months but may be as long as one year. Complications such as neoplastic change are rare and the main problem with warts is that in some cases cure is difficult to achieve and the recurrence rate is high.

Molluscum contagiosum is a harmless skin condition caused by a large pox virus. The diagnosis is usually clinically obvious and the incubation period is between two weeks and three months.

Of the two infestations, scabies is less common than pediculosis pubis. Scabies, however, is usually more troublesome than the latter, itching being the main symptom. It is not as a rule experienced until the patient has become sensitised to some products of the acarus, which may be 4 – 6 weeks after the disease was contracted and it may be slow to subside after treatment. The most commonly affected sites are the interdigital clefts and the ulnar border of the wrists, but the whole body from the head down may be affected, including the genitalia. Pubic lice, as opposed to head and body lice, are generally sexually transmitted but may occasionally be acquired from fomites. Pubic lice may sometimes affect the hair of the chest and axillae. While pruritis may occur, the infestation is often present without the patient being aware of it. The intensity of the itching is dependent upon the host's hypersensitivity to mite antigens.

Recently the acquired immunodeficiency syndrome (AIDS) has been described. It has been found in both sexes, although predominantly in homosexual men. Its aetiology and mode of transmission are unknown although studies have suggested that sexual transmission may be the case in some instances. While some patients are extremely ill due to rare opportunistic infections, such as *Pneumocystis carinii* pneumonia, others develop the rare malignant skin condition, Kaposi's sarcoma.

Warts

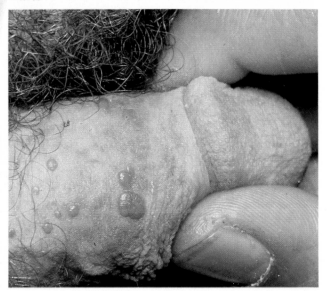

Fig. 159 Warts on the penis are usually multiple, and on the shaft are often flat and keratinised. This type of lesion does not respond well to topical therapy.

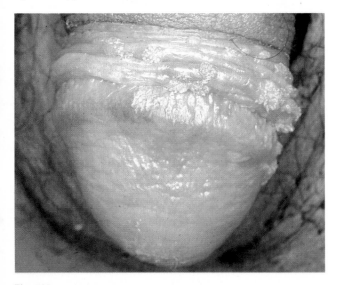

Fig. 160 In the moister subpreputial area, warts are often exophytic and tend to respond well to topical applications.

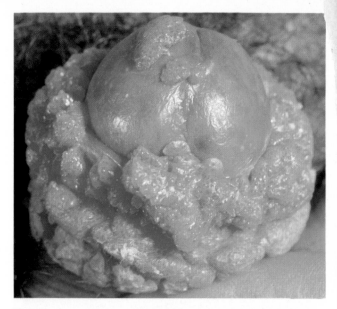

Fig. 161 In the moist conditions of the subpreputial area, the lesions can sometimes proliferate and enlarge markedly. Treatment may be facilitated if other sexually transmitted diseases are diagnosed and treated, as a urethral discharge can maintain subpreputial moistness.

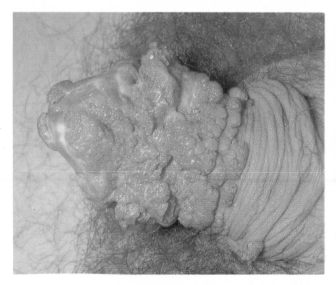

Fig. 162 Sometimes warts can proliferate and enlarge to the extent that the normal anatomy may be distorted.

89

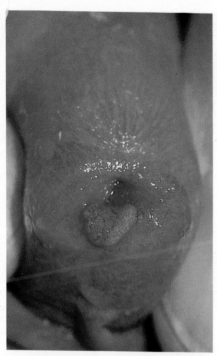

Fig. 163 The urethral meatus is a common site for warts. Sometimes lesions may extend further down the urethra than the fossa navicularis. Urethral and meatal warts can be associated with a urethral discharge.

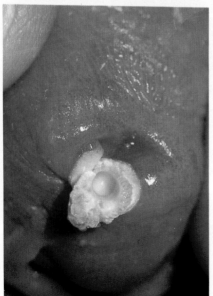

Fig. 164 A frozen meatal wart. Treatment of meatal warts with topical applications can occasionally result in scarring and narrowing of the meatus. Cryotherapy is the treatment of choice.

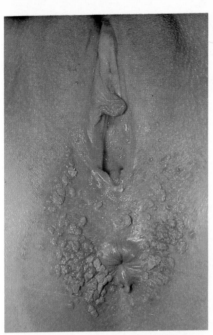

Fig. 165 Perianal warts can occur in both sexes and, because of the moist nature of the area, may proliferate and enlarge.

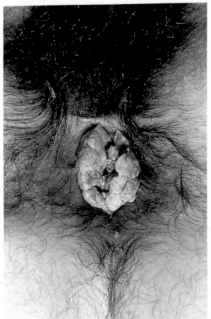

Fig. 166 Large perianal lesions are not unusual, and in the keratinised form, can present a problem with therapy.

91

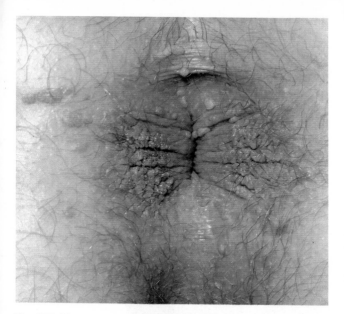

Fig. 167 Warts may be found in the perianal area and can often extend into the anal canal.

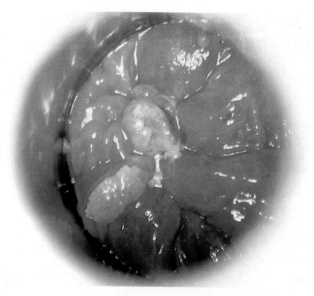

Fig. 168 Lesions can sometimes be found in the rectum. When a patient with perianal warts is examined, a proctoscope should always be passed to exclude anal canal and rectal lesions.

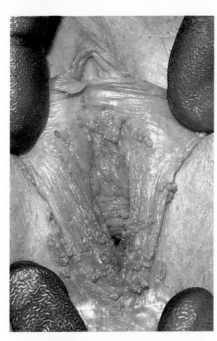

Fig. 169 Multiple small exophytic growths are often found in the vulvo-perineal area. They can enlarge dramatically as the area is moist and can extend into the vagina.

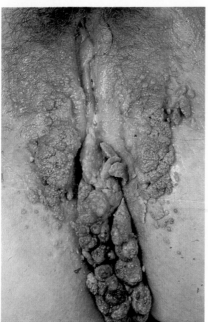

Fig. 170 When warts are extensive in the female genital area, the vulval, perineal and perianal areas are often affected together. It is always wise to exclude other concomitant genital infections.

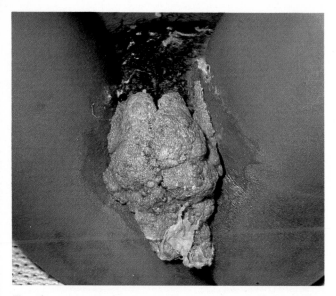

Fig. 171 In the pregnant state, genital warts can enlarge dramatically and can occasionally cause obstruction of labour. They are very difficult to treat in pregnancy but often regress substantially afterwards.

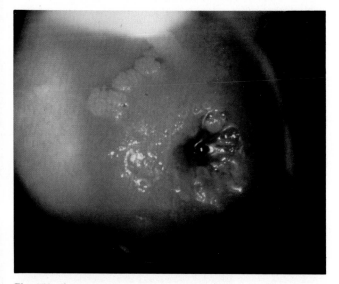

Fig. 172 Recent work has shown that cervical warts are not always visible with the naked eye, but may require colposcopic examination to reveal them. The wart virus may be a factor in subsequent cervical cellular abnormalities.

94

Infestations

SCABIES

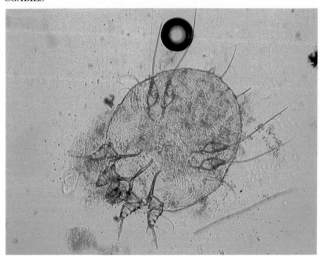

Fig. 173 Scabies is caused by the mite, *Sarcoptes scabiei*. It is transmitted during close bodily contact so it is often sexually acquired. The acarus may be removed from the skin by scraping a burrow with a blunt blade or scarifier and examining the scrapings as a wet preparation with 20% potassium hydroxide.

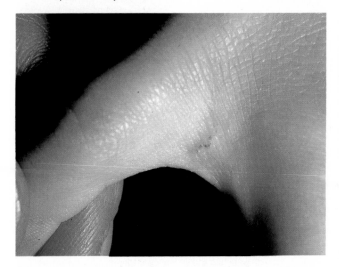

Fig. 174 Although scabetic lesions may be quite widespread, it is not always easy to find a burrow. However, the interdigital spaces and the wrist are commonly affected sites where burrows may be seen.

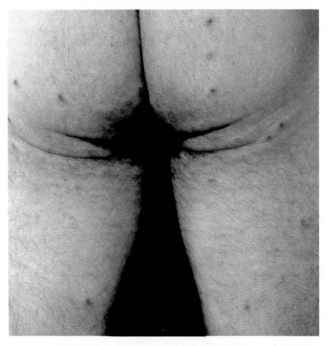

Fig. 175 Scabetic lesions of the buttocks and thighs.

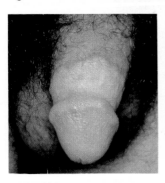

Fig. 176 The genital area can certainly also be affected, and penile lesions, as seen here, are not uncommon. The lesions are less common on the external genitalia of women. Other sexually transmissible diseases should be excluded in cases of genital scabies.

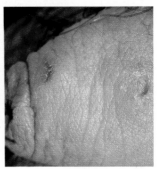

Fig. 177 This close-up shows typical scabetic lesions of the prepuce, although any part of the penis and scrotum can be affected. There is always a tendency to scratch, especially in the genital region and pruritis may persist for some time, certainly weeks in some cases, despite treatment.

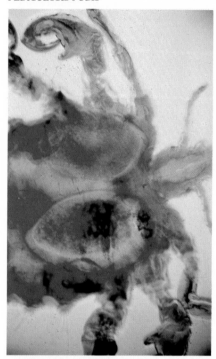

Fig. 178 Pediculosis pubis or 'crabs' is caused by the crab-louse, *Phthirius pubis*, seen in this low power photomicrograph. The lice mate and lay their eggs on the pubic hairs where they are firmly cemented. New adults develop within 2-3 weeks. Pubic lice, as opposed to head and body lice, are generally sexually acquired.

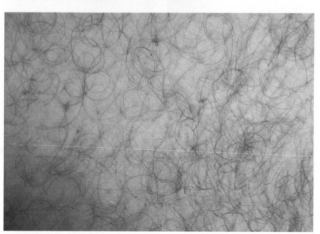

Fig. 179 It is sometimes difficult to visualise pediculosis pubis with the naked eye, especially in dark-skinned people. Careful routine inspection of the pubic hair will usually reveal the condition. A small magnifying glass is helpful. In this case lice and nits are visible.

Molluscum contagiosum

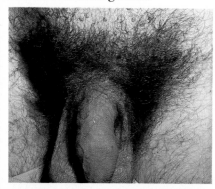

Fig. 180 Molluscum contagiosum can be found anywhere on the body and is transmitted by close bodily contact. Lesions in the genital area or, as here, in one of the most commonly affected areas, the pubic region, imply spread by sexual contact. Note that a penile lesion is also visible.

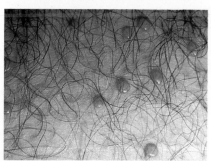

Fig. 181 When examined closely the lesions are seen to be flesh-coloured and waxy. The papules are raised with a central depression from which it is possible to express a soft, cheese-like material. They may become secondarily infected and appear pustular.

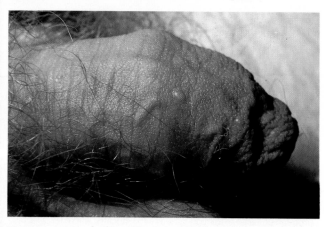

Fig. 182 When sexually acquired, lesions are most often found in the pubic area, or the inner thighs but also on the genitalia – the penis in this case. The vulva may also be affected. Symptoms are few unless there is secondary infection, but mild irritation or pruritis is sometimes described.

Kaposi's sarcoma

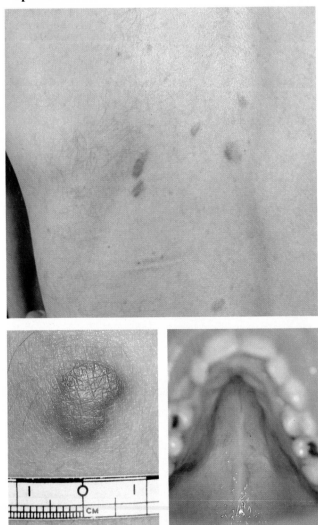

Fig. 183 Kaposi's sarcoma may develop in some patients with AIDS. Whereas previously most cases seen were in elderly people of eastern European or Italian extraction, as well as in Africans, where lesions tended to be on the lower limbs, with AIDS the lesions are occurring at any site on the body and they are often multiple. Well-developed skin lesions often have a pigmented ring around them (left), and some patients have lesions on the palate (right) as well as further down the gastro-intestinal tract.

Index

Entries in **bold** refer to Fig. numbers

Abscess
  Bartholin's duct, **50**
  in granuloma inguinale,
  157
  in lymphogranuloma
  venereum, **150**
  periurethral, **21, 51**
Acquired immunity
deficiency syndrome
(AIDS), 87, **183**
Alopecia in secondary
syphilis, **112-4**
Aneurysms, syphilis and,
123-5
Anus
  primary syphilis, **78**
  secondary syphilis, **101**
  warts, **165-8, 170**
Aorta, effects of syphilis,
123
Arthritis
  Reiter's disease, **5**
  septic gonococcal, **27**
Arthropathy, Charcot's,
127, 128

Balanitis
  candidal, **33**
  circinate, **6, 7, 34**
  plasma cell, of Zoon, 34
  and ulceration, 33, 34
Balanoposthitis, 3
  in NSU, **2**
Bartholin's duct
  abscess, **50**
  discharge from, **49**
Behçet's disease, 33, 34

Bejal, **136**
Bone lesions in tertiary
syphilis, **122**
Brain, effects of syphilis
on, **126**
Bubo
  in chancroid, **144**
  in lymphogranuloma
  venereum, **146, 148,
  149**
  pseudo-, **157**
Buccal mucosa
  Reiter's disease, **8**
  secondary syphilis, **107**

*Calymmatobacterium
granulomatis*, **153**
Candida
  and balanitis, **33**, 33, 34
  and posthitis, 34
  and urethritis, 3, 4, **34**
Candida albicans, **28**
Candidosis
  balanitis and, 33, 34
  primary cutaneous, of
  vulva, **30**
  vaginal (thrush), **28,
  29, 32**
  discharge in, 19, 20, **32**
Carcinoma
  of tongue, **121**
  ulceration and, 34
Cervicitis, 20
  gonococcal, **47**
  non-specific, 20, **42**
Cervix
  ectopy, 19, 20

follicles on, **42**
herpesvirus and, **60**
infections, 19, 20
neoplasms, 19, 20
polyps, 20
syphilis, **77, 110**
warts, **172**
Chancres, **65-83**
Chancroid, 33, 34, **137-44**
Charcot's arthropathy, **127, 128**
Chlamydia trachomatis, **1**
cervicitis, 20, **42**
ophthalmia neonatorum, **45, 46**
pneumonia, **46**
rectal infection, **43, 44**
urethritis, **3, 4,** 4
Clue cells, **39**
Condylomata accuminata (genital warts), 87, **105, 159-72**
Condylomata lata, **101-6**
Conjunctivitis
gonococcal infection, **24**
Reiter's disease, **9**
Cornea, scarring of, **133**
Crabs *see* Pediculosis pubis
Crystalluria, 3, 4

Deafness in congenital syphilis, **133**
Dementia, syphilis and, **126**
Donovania granulomatis, **153**
Drug eruptions, 33, 34
Dyspareunia in trichomoniasis, **38**
Dysuria, herpesvirus infection and, **56**

Elephantiasis in lymphogranuloma

venereum, **150-2**
Endocarditis, gonococcal, **27**
Epididymitis in gonorrhoea, **19**
Erythroplasia of Queyrat, 34
Escherichia coli urethritis, 3
Eyelid, chancre, **83**
Eyes
chlamydial infection, **45, 46**
congenital syphilis, **133**
gonococcal infection, **24, 52**
Reiter's disease, **9**

Fasciitis in Reiter's disease, **5**
Feet
neurosyphilis, **129**
Reiter's disease, **12, 13**
secondary syphilis, **97, 98**
Fingers
chancre, **81**
herpes, **63**
Furuncle, ruptured, 34

Gardnerella vaginalis, **39**
vaginal discharge, 19, 20, **40, 41**
General paralysis of the insane (GPI), **126**
Glands
infection in gonorrhoea, **20, 21**
see also lymphadenitis; lymphadenopathy; lymphogranuloma venereum
Glossitis, chronic superficial, **120**
Gonococcus *see Neisseria*

gonorrhoeae
Gonorrhoea, 3, 4, **17-27, 47, 52**
Granuloma inguinale, 33, 34, **153-8**
Groove-sign, **147, 148**
Gumma, **115-22, 134, 135**

Haemophilus ducreyi, **137**
Hair loss in syphilis, **112-14**
Hands
  scabies, **174**
  secondary syphilis, **97, 99, 100**
  see also fingers
Herpes
  genital, 33, 34, **53-61, 76**
  perianal, **62**
  urethritis, 3, 4
  whitlow, **63**
Herpes hominis virus, 20
Hutchinson's triad, **133**
Hydrocele in gonorrhoea, **19**

Joints
  gonorrhoea, **25, 27**
  Reiter's disease, **5**
  syphilis, **127, 128**

Kaposi's sarcoma, 87, **183**
Keratitis, interstitial, **133**
Keratoderma blennorrhagica, **12, 13**
Klebsiella urethritis, 3

Labia majora, syphilis of, **75**
Labia minora
  herpes, **57**
  syphilis, **73**
Larynx, secondary

syphilis, **107**
Leukoplakia, **120, 121**
Lice, pubic, 87, **178-9**
Littré's glands in gonorrhoea, **21**
Lymphadenitis in chancroid, **144**
Lymphadenopathy
  generalised, in secondary syphilis, **111**
  inguinal
    granuloma inguinale, **157**
    primary syphilis and, **72**
    tropical ulcers and, 33
Lymphogranuloma venereum, 33, 34, **145-52**

Meatitis in NSU, **2, 3**
Meatus, urethral
  chancre at, **71**
  follicles at, in NSU, **4**
  herpesvirus infection, **56**
  pouting of, in NSU, **2**
  warts, 3, **163-4**
Meningitis, gonococcal, **27**
Molluscum contagiosum, 87, **180-2**
Mouth lesions
  Kaposi's sarcoma, **183**
  Reiter's disease, **8**
  syphilis
    congenital, **131, 132, 134**
    primary, **79, 80**
    secondary, **106**
    tertiary, **119, 120**
Mucous membrane lesions
  Reiter's disease, **8**
  secondary syphilis, **107-10**

tertiary syphilis, **118, 119**

Neisseria gonorrhoeae, **14-16**
  infections, **17-21**
    cervical, 20, **47**
    disseminated, **22-7, 52**

Neoplasms
  cervical, 19, 20
  ulceration and, 33, 34
  see also carcinoma; sarcoma

Neurosyphilis, **126-9**

Non-specific urethritis (NSU), 3, 4

Ophthalmia neonatorum
  chlamydial, **45, 46**
  gonococcal, **52**

Palate
  Kaposi's sarcoma, **183**
  perforated, **134**

Papillomavirus, 87

Pediculosis pubis, 87, **178-9**

Penis
  chancroid, **137-41**
  elephantiasis, **150**
  granuloma inguinale, **153, 154, 158**
  herpes, **53-6**
  infestations, **177**
  molluscum contagiosum, **180-2**
  'saxophone', **150**
  syphilis
    primary, **65-72**
    secondary, **90, 106, 109**
  warts, **159-62**
  see also balanitis

Perihepatitis, gonococcal, **27**

Perineum, warts, **169, 170**

Pharyngitis, gonococcal, **23**

Pharynx, secondary syphilis, **107**

Phthirius pubis, **178**

Pinta, **136**

Pneumocystis carinii pneumonia, 87

Polyarthralgia in gonorrhoea, **25**

Posthitis
  candidal, **34**
  Reiter's disease, **7**

Prepuce
  chancroid, **139**
  herpes, **54**
  infestations, **177**
  inflammation *see* posthitis
  primary syphilis, **68, 69**
  secondary syphilis, **109**
  warts, **160-2**

Proctitis, herpetic, **62**

Prostatitis in gonorrhoea, **19**

Prostatorrhoea, 3, 4

Proteus urethritis, 3

Pruritus
  in candidosis, **29, 30**
  in infestations, 87, **177**
  molluscum contagiosum, **182**
  vulval, 20, **36, 38**

Queyrat, erythroplasia of, 34

Rectum
  chlamydial infection, **43, 44**
  gonorrhoea of, **22**
  herpetic infection, **62**
  warts, **168**

Reiter's disease, **5-11**
  balanitis in, 33, 34
Rhagades, **131**

Salpingitis, 20
Sarcoma, Kaposi's, 87,
183
Sarcoptes scabiei, **173**
Scabies, 33, 34, 87, **173-7**
Scrotum
  elephantiasis, **151**
  gonorrhoea, **19**
  infestations, **177**
  in syphilis, **52, 106**
Skin
  gonococcal infection,
  25, 26
  Kaposi's sarcoma, 87,
  183
  secondary syphilis, **84-100**
  tertiary syphilis, **115-6**
Smegma, 3
Soft sore (chancroid), 33,
34, **137-44**
Spine, effects of syphilis,
125, 127, 128
Stevens Johnson syndrome,
34
Syphilide, **84-100**
  annular, **96**
  corymbose, **95**
  nodular cutaneous, **115**
  papulo-pustular, **93, 94**
  papulo-squamous, **92**
Syphilis
  cardiovascular, **123-5**
  congenital, 72, **130-5**
  endemic, **136**
  neuro-, **126-9**
  primary, **65-83**
  secondary, **84-113**
  tertiary (gummatous),
  64, **115-22, 134, 135**

  ulceration in, 33, 34
Syphilitic snuffles, **130**

Tabes dorsalis, **127, 129**
Teeth
  congenital syphilis, **132**
  Hutchinson's, **132**
Tendinitis, Reiter's
disease, **5**
Throat lesions
  secondary syphilis,
  107, 109
  tertiary syphilis, **118**
Thrush *see* candidosis,
vaginal
Tibia
  sabre, **122**
  tertiary syphilis, **122**
Tongue
  carcinoma, **121**
  in Reiter's disease, **8**
  syphilis
    primary, **79**
    secondary, **106**
    tertiary, **120, 121**
Treponema pallidum, **64**
Trichomonas vaginalis, **35**
  urethritis, 3, 4, **38**
  vaginitis, 19, **37**
    discharge in, **36**
Two-glass test, **18**
Tyson's glands in
gonorrhoea, **20**

Ulcers
  genital,
    tropical, 33, 34
    tuberculous, 34
  perforating, **129**
  snail-trail, **108**
Urethra
  discharge from, 3
    in gonorrhoea, **17, 48**
    in herpesvirus
    infection, **36**

in NSU, **2, 3**
   warts and, **163**
stricture of, 3
warts, 3, **163**
Urethritis, 3, 4
   anterior, **18**
   chemical, 3
   non-specific (NSU), 3, 4
      urethral discharge in,
      2
   posterior, **18**
   see also gonorrhoea *and*
   specific organisms
Urine retention,
herpesvirus infection and,
56, 59, 62

Vagina
   candidosis, **28, 29**
   discharge from, 19-20
      in candidosis, **32**
      Gardnerella vaginalis,
      40, 41
      gonococcal cervicitis,
      47, 49
      non-specific cervicitis,
      42
      in trichomoniasis, **36,
      37**
   wall, secondary syphilis,
   110
Vaginitis
   bacterial, 20
   post-menopausal, 19, 20
   trichomonal, **37**
Vincent's organisms, 34
Vulva
   chancroid, **143**
   elephantiasis, **152**
   herpes, **57-61, 76**
   molluscum contagiosum,
   98
   primary cutaneous
   candidosis, **30, 31**
   pruritus, 20, **36, 38**

syphilis
   primary, **73-7**
   secondary, **101, 104,
   110**
warts, **169-71**
Vulvitis, trichomonal, **38**

Warts, genital
(condylomata accuminata),
3, 87, **105, 159-72**
Whitlow, herpetic, **63**

Yaws, **136**